W9-BBM-609

Nature's *Best*

HERBAL REMEDIES

Sure Cures for More Than
75 Common Health Problems
from America's Most Respected
Herb Doctor

JAMES A. DUKE, Ph.D.

Rodale Press, Inc.
Emmaus, Pennsylvania

Notice

This book is meant to increase your knowledge of the latest developments in the use of plants for medicinal purposes. Because everyone is different, a physician must diagnose conditions and supervise the use of healing herbs to treat individual health problems. Herbs and other natural remedies are not substitutes for professional medical care. We urge you to seek the best medical resources available to help you make informed decisions.

The information in this book is excerpted from *The Green Pharmacy* (Rodale Press, 1997).

© 1999 by James A. Duke
Cover photograph © 1999 by Anthony Loew

All rights reserved. No part of this publication may be reproduced or transmitted in any form or by any means, electronic or mechanical, including photocopying, recording, or any other information storage and retrieval system, without the written permission of the publisher.

Printed in the United States of America on acid-free ∞, recycled paper ♻

Cover Designer: Richard Kershner

ISBN 1–57954–254–9 paperback

Distributed to the book trade by St. Martin's Press

2   4   6   8   10   9   7   5   3   paperback

Visit us on the Web at www.preventionbookshelf.com, or call us toll-free at (800) 848-4735.

─── OUR PURPOSE ───

We inspire and enable people to improve
their lives and the world around them.

Introduction

This book is the culmination of many decades of work with medicinal plants throughout the world and many years of plant-hunting, from China to Costa Rica, from Peru to Pennsylvania, from the hills of Virginia to the upper reaches of the Amazon.

For most of my 35-year career, I worked for the U.S. Department of Agriculture (USDA) as a botanist specializing in medicinal plants. Technically, I'm what is known as an ethnobotanist, which simply means that I've studied how plants are used as food and medicine in many different cultures. During my career, I've personally seen medicinal herbs successfully treat conditions that high-tech pharmaceuticals could scarcely touch.

In part 1 of this book, you'll find my advice about finding, preparing, and even growing herbs. You'll also find my advice and safety cautions about using them. These are based on personal experiences as well as an extensive database of scientific information about the various chemicals and compounds found in plants.

In part 2, I have applied a rating system of sorts to highlight the herbs and herbal remedies that I believe to be the most effective for each of the diseases and health problems. The most highly recommended herbs have a three-star ★★★ rating. For alternate remedies, however, be sure to pay attention to herbs with two-star ★★ and one-star ★ ratings.

Contents

PART 1

Herbs: Nature's Amazing Medicines

PART 2

A Practical Guide to the Best Herbal Remedies

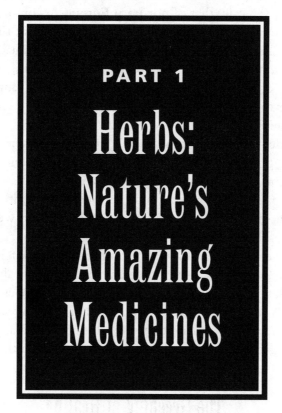

PART 1

Herbs: Nature's Amazing Medicines

What Is an Herb, Anyway?

If you're reading this book, you probably know what an herb is . . . or do you? The term *herb* should be easy to define, but actually, it's surprisingly difficult.

The classic botanical definition is that an herb is a nonwoody plant that dies down to its roots each winter. Clearly, this definition was concocted by botanists in a cold climate, specifically that of northern Europe. According to this definition, there are no herbs in the Amazonian rain forest, one of the world's most botanically diverse, herb-rich habitats, because there is no winter.

The classic definition also excludes woody trees and shrubs, including ginkgo and hawthorn, two of the biggest-selling medicinal "herbs" in Europe. That's why some people prefer the term *botanicals* (and *botanical medicine*): It includes trees and shrubs as well as herbs.

Using a broader definition, some people consider an herb to be simply a useful plant. The big problem with this definition is that in one very important sense, all green plants are useful, even those that are not food and have no place in medicine or commerce. All green plants perform photosynthesis, combining sunlight, carbon dioxide and water and releasing the oxygen we all breathe. I'd say that's pretty useful.

For the purposes of this book, I define an herb simply as a medicinal plant. It can be woody or nonwoody, from a cold climate or a tropical one. It can be a wild or tame food, a weed, a culinary spice or whatever. It doesn't even have to be green. Plenty of barks, roots and plant parts that are not green are medicinal and therefore are included here. And there are a lot of medicinal mushrooms out there that are not green and that do deserve more attention than they'll get in this book.

The Greening of Healing

Most Americans believe that we have the best health-care system in the world—at least that's what all the doctors and government health experts keep trying to tell us. But anyone who has ever gotten the run-around from a doctor or had to deal with a health insurance company knows that if what we have is the best, then the best still leaves a lot to be desired.

Most Americans assume that the pharmaceuticals their doctors prescribe are unquestionably better than the herbal medicines that few doctors and relatively few Americans know much about. It delights me to no end that this picture is changing rapidly.

I've been a botanist specializing in medicinal plants for most of my 35-year career, and I've personally seen medicinal herbs successfully treat conditions that high-tech pharmaceuticals could not touch.

The reason herbs are not more popular in the United States is that the drug companies can't patent them. The drug companies make their money by pulling the medicinally active molecules out of herbs and then tinkering with them a little until they're chemically unique. The companies can then patent their new molecules, give them brand names and sell them back to us for a lot more money than their original herbal sources cost.

Herbs Are Good Medicine

Of course, the drug companies always say that their unique molecules are better, stronger, more targeted and safer than herbs. I'll readily agree that they are stronger. In fact, they're often too strong and have bad side effects that their herbal precursors might not have.

As for pharmaceuticals being better, that's sometimes hard to say. In some studies, herbal products clearly perform better. Ginger, for example, has been shown to be superior to pharmaceutical dimenhydrate (Dramamine) as a preventive therapy for motion sickness.

I'm not saying that pharmaceuticals are bad. I am saying that we need more research that tests herbs against pharmaceutical drugs. Until that happens, we simply won't know which is better. That leads me to the rather shocking conclusion that Americans are not necessarily getting the best medicine. Herbal therapies may, in many cases, prove to be more economical, more effective and safer—all with fewer side effects—than the pharmaceuticals.

Our challenge is to transcend the assumptions that are made by doctors, the advertising and promotion of the drug companies and the narrow and restrictive drug approval process used by the U.S. government. Our challenge is to think green—not the mercenary, monetary green of the pharmaceutical firms but the cleansing, empowering green of chlorophyll, the green that feeds, fuels, oxygenates and medicates our planet.

Economics drives the pharmaceutical companies, but what drives herbal medicine and the "green lifestyle" in general is ecology, the idea that we're connected to everything else on the planet and that we all thrive or fall together.

Putting Safety First

I'll be the first to admit that herbal medicine is not risk-free. To benefit from using herbs, you need to have some basic background information. Then you need to have confidence in the herbs you use and in any herbal practitioner you consult. This is no different from conventional medicine, where you need to have confidence in your physician and any pharmaceutical you take.

As a rule, however, rational herbal medicine is safer than conventional medicine because the herbal medicines are more dilute and side effects tend to be less severe.

But you still have to exercise caution when using herbal medicines. You also need to understand that things can go wrong. There are a number of strategies that you can use to protect yourself.

First of all, get the right stuff. Unless you are absolutely sure of an herb's identity, don't take it. This rule applies mainly to people who are picking herbs in the wild, of course. People have been known to eat poisonous or dangerous plants simply because they misidentified an herb and took something other than what they thought they were taking. The classic killer is poison hemlock, which looks rather like wild parsley or wild parsnip.

The Universe of Herbs

While there are some 300,000 higher plant species that are all chemically distinct, fewer than 10 percent of them have been carefully screened for their medicinal and toxic constituents. A really good herbalist might know 1,000 to 2,000 species, rarely more.

This means that experienced as well as inexperienced herbalists can make mistakes. Not too long ago, while gathering herbs for a weekend class in the Blue Ridge Mountains, yours truly got all excited at the discovery of some "wild ginseng." Later, on closer examination, I was chagrined to discover that the supposed ginseng was Virginia creeper.

Of course, herbalists are not alone in making the occasional error. Physicians and pharmacists make them as well. And I personally feel safer consulting a well-informed herbalist than I do consulting most doctors. As for the perils of pharmaceuticals, read the fine print on labels or in the advertisements.

As for the identities of commercially packaged herbal products, especially those that are chemically standardized, you can usually trust the labels. But even with standardized extracts, as with pharmaceuticals, there is a very small but still real chance for error.

Watching Out for Problems

Whatever herb you're taking, I recommend that you learn as much as you can about what to expect from it. If anything unexpected happens, stop taking whatever it is and check with an expert you trust.

In addition, here's some further advice for anyone using herbal medicine.

Make sure of the diagnosis. Herbal devotees sometimes get the idea that they can diagnose illness as well as come up with herbs to treat it. But diagnosis is a separate art and one that is best left to physicians. I discourage self-diagnosis.

Diagnosing illness is not easy, and sometimes even good doctors make mistakes. But physicians' diagnostic batting average is usually better than that of anyone who has not had medical training. Once you're confident of a diagnosis, then you can discuss with your physician how to treat it: drugs, herbs, some combination of the two or any of the foregoing plus diet, exercise and lifestyle changes. Some holistic physicians will stress diet and lifestyle more than drugs for some ailments.

Watch out for side effects. I'm convinced that all medicines, natural or synthetic, have side effects. It's hard to imagine an active plant chemical (phytochemical)—or an herbal mixture containing thousands of them—having just one targeted chemical reaction in our body. Of course we have other reactions, unrelated to the illness, that could appropriately be termed side effects—some desirable and some undesirable. That's why you have to watch yourself when taking any new herb for the first time.

If you have an unpleasant reaction to an herb, such as dizziness, nausea or headache, cut back on your dosage or stop taking the herb. Listen to your body. If the herb doesn't feel right, don't take it.

Be alert for allergic reactions. People can be allergic to anything. Even if you have no known allergies, you might be allergic to a new herb that you try. Be careful. Again, listen to your body. If you develop any unusual symptoms, stop taking the herb and consult an allergist or physician.

If you experience any difficulty breathing within 30 minutes or so of trying a new herb, food or drug, call 911 immediately. You may be having an anaphylactic reaction, the most severe form of allergic reaction, which can prove rapidly fatal unless treated promptly.

Anaphylactic reactions to herbs are rare, and I'm not saying that you need to be unduly apprehensive about trying new things. Just be careful and understand the possible risks.

Beware of interactions. Pharmaceutical medicines sometimes interact badly with each other and with certain foods. The same goes for herbal medicines, although many herbal reference books neglect to mention this. Always be particularly careful when taking more than one drug or herb or a combination of a drug and an herb. Bad interactions are always possible. If you suspect a bad interaction, consult your physician or pharmacist.

Here's one interaction that you should be particularly aware of: Antidepressants known as monoamine oxidase (MAO) inhibitors interact badly with wine, cheese and many other foods. If you take a pharmaceutical MAO inhibitor, you shouldn't eat these foods.

The antidepressant herb St.-John's-wort is also an MAO inhibitor, so the same food restrictions apply. If you take St.-John's-wort regularly, consult a physician, pharmacist or consumer drug guide about which foods to avoid.

Open lines of communication. Too many people listen to both their physicians and their herbalists and do what both advise. Usually there's no problem with this, such as when a physician gives you sleeping pills for insomnia, for example, and an herbalist recommends a hot bath before bed with a blend of sedative aromatherapy oils.

But just as too many cooks can spoil the broth, too many health practitioners can also be too much of a good thing. Let's say your physician prescribes an MAO inhibitor for depression, and your herbalist recommends St.-John's-wort, also an MAO inhibitor. You may wind up taking too much. Or let's say your physician prescribes half an aspirin a day to prevent heart attack, and your herbalist tells you to drink a daily cup of tea made from willow bark or wintergreen. The teas contain the herbal equivalent of aspirin, and you might wind up taking more than you need, with more anti-clotting action than you want.

To avoid the too-many-cooks problem, be sure to tell your physician and your herbalist about *all* the medicines you're taking as well as any unusual foods you might be eating.

A Word to Wise Moms-to-Be

As a general rule, women shouldn't take herbs while they're pregnant unless they discuss their selections with their obstetricians first.

There's a good reason for this. Quite a few herbs can increase the risk of miscarriage. Maine herbalist Deb Soule, author of the feminist herbal *The Roots of Healing*, advises pregnant women to avoid the following herbs: barberry root bark, cascara sagrada, feverfew, juniper berries, mugwort, pennyroyal, pokeroot, rue, senna, southernwood, tansy, thuja, and wormwood. That sounds like good advice to me, and I would add a few more to this list: balsam pear, chervil, Chinese angelica, hernandia, hyptis, mayapple and mountain mint. Lately I've also seen caution flags about evening primrose and St.-John's-wort, but I haven't seen the rationale behind these caveats.

It's also a good idea not to binge on celery or parsley. Eating a little of these healthy vegetables won't do any harm, but eating a lot could conceivably cause a problem.

If you're a woman who's pregnant, you should limit your consumption of caffeine as well. One study showed what the researchers called a "strong association of caffeine intake during pregnancy and fetal loss." As little as 163 milligrams of caffeine per day—the amount in one to two cups of brewed coffee—might double the risk of spontaneous abortion.

In addition, here are a few more "don'ts" during pregnancy: Don't smoke, don't drink alcohol, and again, don't take any drugs, including over-the-counter products, except on the advice of your physician.

Buying and Harvesting Medicinal Herbs

Are you interested in herbal medicines, but you're not quite sure how to get started? Never fear—the information in this book will help you, whether you're an herbal neophyte just taking the first steps or someone who already uses herbs on a regular basis.

The chapters in part 2 of this book will tell you which herbs you need to prevent and treat specific diseases. But before you ever use your first herb, you need to know how to obtain them.

There are, in fact, several ways to get the herbs that I discuss in this book. Many you can buy, but there are some that you may want to plant, harvest and process yourself.

It's quicker, easier and sometimes safer and surer to simply buy herbal medicines, but in doing so, you forgo the exercise and miss the spiritual power of planting, nurturing, harvesting, processing and preparing your own green medicines. I'm an avid gardener. If you are, too, you know the joy it brings. But the important thing is to go green on any level that suits you.

Buying Standardized Medicinal Herbs

It is perfectly acceptable to buy what are known as standardized herbal products at a health food store or herb shop. In fact, these herbal preparations are gaining in popularity so rapidly that there's a good chance you'll even be able to find many of them at your local drugstore.

Standardized means that the herbal products have been processed a bit to guarantee a known minimum level of one or more of the major active ingredients. These products are the best quality you can purchase. Standardization largely compensates for the natural variability you find in bulk herbs—the kind available in bins or jars and measured out according to weight—and it takes the uncertainty out of herbal preparations. You know exactly how much of the active ingredients you're getting.

Unfortunately, standardization makes herbs more expensive than the bulk herb would be. Even so, these "expensive" standardized herbal extracts are still only about a tenth as costly, on average, as the pharmaceuticals that treat the same conditions, so you're still way ahead when you take the standardized green route.

Standardized extracts do vary somewhat, because the longer these herbal medicines are stored, the less potent they become. But then, pharmaceuticals are not perfect either.

You can usually find standardized herbal extracts quite easily wherever herbal products are sold. If you don't see them, ask for them. If an herbal product is standardized, it will say so on the label.

What the Labels Won't Tell You

Unfortunately, the labels of herbal preparations often don't say much else. That's because an herb must be approved as a "drug" in the eyes of the Food and Drug Administration (FDA) in order to specify its medical or therapeutic use. Herb marketers must spend on the order of $200 million proving to the agency's satisfaction that the herb in question is safe and effective enough to justify a medicinal claim. Of course, only the big drug companies have this kind of money, and who in his right mind would spend millions to prove the benefits of a plant no one can patent?

In the same way, manufacturers are prohibited from labeling herb products to specify possible side effects. That's because the FDA views this information as medicinal claims. Without clear labeling, consumers are left largely uninformed.

One purpose of this book, of course, is to provide you with the information that you need in order to use herbs safely and effectively. Nevertheless, I sincerely wish the FDA would allow good information to be included on herb labels. Anyone should have access to this information when they buy an herbal medicine. I hope that if enough of us pester the FDA long enough, perhaps one day we will be able to buy standardized herbs that are well-labeled for consumers.

Here are a dozen very important medicinal herbs that I'd suggest buying as standardized products. (If for any reason you can't buy the standardized products, it's certainly fine to use these—with the exception of ginkgo—as bulk herbs.)

Calendula. Buy it as a salve to treat bruises, cuts and scrapes.

Camomile. A tincture provides a reliable sedative and can be used to make a stomach-settling tea.

Echinacea. The flowers and roots stimulate the immune system to help fight disease.

Evening primrose. This flower produces a valuable seed oil that's too difficult to extract at home.

Ginkgo. This herb comes from a huge tree whose leaves must be processed into a concentrated extract to be medically useful.

Ginseng. The medicinal roots of this plant do not mature for at least five years. It is too complicated to grow and process this plant yourself. (At present, the deer are harvesting my own ginseng patch.)

Hawthorn. This slow-growing shrub is useful for treating heart problems. It's a powerful medicine that should be taken only under a doctor's supervision.

Kava kava. This herb is a safe, mild tranquilizer that grows only in tropical forests.

Licorice. Here's an anti-ulcer herb that is simply too hard to grow, at least where I come from. (This fact comes from someone who has tried several times to grow licorice but has never been successful.)

Milk thistle. The prickly leaves of this herb make it too painful to harvest yourself.

Red pepper. A plant that grows in tropical climates, red pepper contains a potent, pain-relieving compound—capsaicin—that often shows up in standardized products.

Teatree. A tropical plant that will not grow in most of the United States, teatree is an excellent, widely used antiseptic.

Buying Bulk Herbs

I use bulk herbs frequently, picking them by the handful in my six-acre Herbal Vineyard, my home of 25 years in Fulton, Maryland. Along with making teas, I also juice them, and I frequently add them to foods and beverages.

You don't have to be into gardening to get bulk herbs, however. Many health food stores and herb shops have rows of bins of dried bulk herbs that sell for a reasonable price.

There's a downside, however. Whether you buy herbs or grow them yourself, you can never be certain of the levels of active constituents in bulk plant material. This is the main shortcoming of bulk herbal medicines compared with standardized extracts and pharmaceuticals.

The payoff, to my way of thinking, is that using bulk herbs gives you the opportunity to experiment a little more and become more intimate with the plant. This produces a spiritual connection of the kind American Indians have long celebrated. I believe that this spiritual connection is therapeutic. It always has been for me.

But what about safety?

Not to worry. The vast majority of the medicinal herbs discussed in this book are safe even in large doses. And if you need to use special caution with a particular herb or when treating a particular health condition, I let you know in that chapter. So using bulk herbs doesn't really present much of a safety issue. The one concern is that with some batches you might not get enough potency—enough of the active compounds—to give you the therapeutic results you need.

The Variability Factor

Why can't you be sure of the potency of bulk herbs? There are many reasons.

Genetics. Different strains of an herb can have genetic differences in potency. For example, levels of sanguinarine, a biologically active compound found in the antiseptic bloodroot plant, *Sanguinaria*, may vary tenfold based on the genetics of different plants. And variations of a thousandfold or ten thousandfold may occur even within a given species of thyme.

Growing conditions. These affect the overall health and vigor of the plant. Plants grown in poor soil under stressful climate conditions may not have the same potency as plants grown in rich soil under ideal conditions. (Surprisingly, stressed plants often have higher levels of medicinal compounds.)

Timing and method of harvesting. Think of the difference in taste, texture and succulence between immature peaches and ripe peaches. Herbs don't ripen as fruits do, but the concentrations of active constituents vary considerably during their life cycles. For optimal potency, ginseng roots should not be harvested before they are at least five years old, but some growers harvest earlier to rush the roots to market. Those roots won't necessarily contain optimal levels of the active compounds.

Drying. Fresh herbs are most appealing. Just think of the difference between fresh mint and dried mint. Both smell and taste minty, but the fresh leaf is much more aromatic, meaning that it contains more of its medicinal oil. Whenever you smell an herb, it loses a tiny bit of its essence and power because its potency is contained in the aromatic molecules that land on the smell receptors in your nose. Once they leave the plant, they're gone.

Of course, herbs don't stay fresh for very long. That's why the convention among herbalists is to develop recipes using dried herbs, which can be stored fairly easily for many months. But the longer you store the herbs, the less potent they become. Light, oxygen and heat trigger chemical changes that make them lose potency—go stale—over time. That's why most herbalists recommend storing dried herbs in airtight, dark glass containers and keeping them cool. Careful storage greatly extends shelf life.

Packaging. In general, the best way to be sure of preserving an herbal medicine's potency is to buy an alcohol tincture or a glycerin extract. These can remain potent for a year or so. The same cannot be said for herbs in tea bags, powdered herbs or herbal capsules, unless they are guarded by added antioxidants. They are quicker to suffer damage from light, oxygen and heat.

Adding Some Spice

In addition to the many herbs that you can buy in bulk or standardized form, there are many spices that double as medicines. You probably already have some of them in your spice rack. With the exception of capsicum, garlic, ginger and turmeric, they are not available in the United States as standardized extracts and, again with the exception of garlic, most are tropical plants that don't grow well here. So you'll probably have to buy them in bulk or powdered form.

Allspice. This tropical herb has a complex aroma and is useful for indigestion.

Cardamom. An expensive spice, cardamom can be a mild stimulant.

Cinnamon. This common, tasty spice has potent antimicrobial action and can settle an upset stomach.

Cloves. Cloves have proven pain-relieving and antiseptic properties.

Garlic. Deservedly called Russian penicillin, this pungent bulb is useful in preventing our major killers—heart disease and cancer.

Ginger. The world's best nausea preventive, ginger is also useful in treating arthritis.

Red pepper. This native American spice works on pain by three different mechanisms.

Sesame. The seeds of this plant are a great source of antioxidants and other therapeutic chemicals.

Turmeric. This yellow spice shows great promise in treating arthritis and diabetes.

In Search of Wild Medicinals

Foraging for wild herbs is known in botanical lingo as wildcrafting. When you're wildcrafting, of course, you aren't dealing with standardized extracts. But in my humble opinion, the physical and mental exercise of wildcrafting, plus the spiritual connection to the plant and the forest where it grows, provides a therapeutic power that more than compensates for the loss of exactness.

As a botanist, wildcrafting is easy for me. I know my plants well and have been foraging in the wild for more than 60 years. Of course, picking wild medicinal herbs can be hazardous, and you don't want to try it unless you can positively identify the plants you're selecting. (I recall one elderly couple out West who mistook foxglove for comfrey. Unfortunately, foxglove is the source of the heart-stimulating drug digitalis, and it had fatal consequences.)

I advise anyone who is not really familiar with field botany to steer clear of the potential hazards of harvesting wild plants. But if you know what you're doing, in just about any part of the United States you can harvest a bounty of useful medicinal herbs just by stepping out your front door.

If you're not familiar with herbs at first, you can have a good deal of fun finding out more about them. Most metropolitan areas have botanical organizations—museum groups, scout groups, hiking clubs or university extension departments—that offer classes in the identification of local edible and medicinal plants. Take it from a long-time forager: Hiking is much more fun when you can munch your way along the trail.

Growing Your Own, Indoors

Like wildcrafting, growing your own herbs gives you nonstandardized bulk plant material. But it also gives you an even deeper spiritual connection to your medicines than foraging, so I'm all for it.

No matter what you grow, gardening is a therapeutic, self-empowering hobby. And from what we know about mind-body medicine, I'm confident that self-grown herbal medicines should work better than anything store-bought or foraged.

I love my Herbal Vineyard, but you don't need an estate—or even a yard—to grow medicinal herbs. All you need is a kitchen windowsill where you can grow a potted aloe plant—your instant, herbal emergency kit in case of accidental burns. (Just snip off a leaf, slit it open and apply the yellow-green inner leaf gel to the burn.)

There are many other herbs that you can raise on a windowsill or on your back porch. If you're a city dweller, you can find space in a roof garden, courtyard, balcony or fire escape. Quite a few medicinal-culinary species that are native to semi-arid climates will also flourish on sunny kitchen windowsills. Here are some to consider.

Basil. This insect-repelling herb is recommended for treating bad breath and headache.

Chives. Along with their cousins garlic, leeks and onions, chives help prevent cancer and treat high blood pressure.

Dill. This herb is deservedly famous as a remedy for colic and gas.

Fennel. This herb is good for treating upset stomach and indigestion.

Hyssop. Mentioned in the Bible, hyssop contains several antiviral compounds and is useful in treating herpes. (It's also under review as an AIDS therapy.)

Lavender. Some varieties of this lovely herb are loaded with sedative compounds that can penetrate the skin. Toss a handful into your bathwater if you want a nice-smelling way to relax.

Parsley. Best known as a great source of chlorophyll for combating bad breath, parsley is rich in zinc, which is good for men's reproductive health. (Yet more than 90 percent of parsley served in restaurants is thrown away.)

Peppermint. This is a major source of cooling, soothing, stomach-settling menthol.

Rosemary. Rich in antioxidants, this tasty culinary spice may help prevent Alzheimer's disease.

Sage. Sage shares much of the medicinal potential of rosemary.

Savory. Europeans add this herb to bean dishes to reduce flatulence.

Thyme. This is one of the best sources of thymol, an antiseptic, stomach-soothing compound that helps prevent the blood clots that cause heart attack.

Growing an Outdoor Herb Garden

In my Herbal Vineyard, I have some 200 species of herbs, most of them medicinal. During the growing season, one of my great pleasures in life is to stroll the grounds and check on all the plants.

Almost hourly, when I'm spending the day at the computer, I take breaks and visit my herb garden. When I harvest a handful of this or that, I often select mints to make up one of my aromatic beverages, usually hot mint tea on a cool morning or iced mint tea on a hot afternoon.

Growing and loving these herbs is one of the most healthful activities I engage in, and I heartily recommend it.

It would take another book to tell you how to grow all the herbs I discuss in this one. But if you do have garden space, here are the perennial medicinal herbs that I recommend. They flourish in my own garden, and I think they'll do well for anyone who gardens in a temperate climate more or less like Maryland's.

Chasteberry. A perennial flowering shrub, this is a great herb for treating women's problems.

Goldenseal. An antibiotic herb, goldenseal grows best when planted in a shady area.

Lemon balm. Also known as melissa, this weedy antiviral mint has sedative properties. Although it sometimes looks like it has died away, it always comes back.

Mountain mint. An insect-repelling herb that should be more popular among gardeners than it is.

Oregano. Another weedy mint—a great source of antioxidants.

Self-heal. The reputation of this mint as a panacea is only slightly exaggerated.

Spearmint. This herb is about as good as peppermint for settling the stomach.

St.-John's-wort. Simply the best herbal treatment for depression.

Tansy. This herb contains some of the same anti-migraine compounds as feverfew.

Valerian. The roots contain a great anxiety-relieving sedative. But be warned—the tea smells like dirty gym socks.

Wild yam. Many herbalists recommend this herb for women's reproductive health.

Willow. The willow tree's easy-peeling bark contains the herbal version of aspirin.

Harvesting and Storing Herbs

Okay, so you've got a big peppermint patch, or whatever, growing in your garden or on your windowsill. Now what?

First you must harvest your herbs. You can snip off leaves and use them as needed. Taking a cue from the American Indians, the romantics among us like to thank the herb for serving us and apologize for mutilating it.

Down in Panama and Peru, I listened as Indian shamans sang long chants to the herbs they were about to harvest, often while facing the East. When I'm not in a hurry, I remember that the plants, too, have lives, and that their lives sustain ours.

In fact, the more we clip the leaves of medicinal plants, the more medicinal they become. This makes sense botanically because herbs' medicinal constituents are basically part of the plant's self-protection system. Harvesting the leaves makes the plant respond as if it's under attack (which it is), so it produces more of what protects it. Studies have shown that infections, insect infestations and leaf-plucking, among other attacks on the plant, increase the levels of some of the same chemicals that we view as medicines.

Collection Times

Although some herbalists argue for harvesting herbs early in the morning while there is still dew on them, I disagree. That dilutes the herb with water, meaning that it has proportionately more water and less chemical until it's dried. In my view, you get the greatest concentration of plant chemicals and the least water when you collect leaves during a hot, dry day, but before the leaves have wilted.

Roots are best collected in spring or fall. Bark may be collected in spring, especially if the compounds you seek are in the living bark. If you're collecting seeds for food, I recommend that you get them before they have dried out and hardened. But if you're harvesting them to plant next year rather than to use immediately, you may want to wait until they've dried out.

Feel free to use herbs fresh, especially in cooking. Fresh culinary herbs and spices almost always taste best. You can also freeze them, dry them or use them to make tinctures. (When harvesting fresh culinary herbs, I generally use a plastic bag to help retain the moisture.)

Preserving the Goods

If you intend to preserve your herbs for future use, it's cheaper to dry them. Collect them in a brown paper bag rather than a plastic bag, and write the name of the plant and the collection date on the outside of the bag.

If you don't stuff it too tightly, many herbs can be dried right in the bag. I always make a run through my herb garden with paper bags before the last killing frost, collecting herbs for my winter medicines, soups and teas.

Check your brown-bagged herbs after about a week, and if they are not clearly drying—becoming papery and crumbly—spread them out on newspapers or clean wood or screen in a dry, shaded area so that they can dry before mildew attacks.

When it comes to success in drying, a great deal depends on your local weather conditions. In arid weather, herbs may dry too rapidly, especially in direct sunlight. In humid and especially in foggy weather, you may have to apply heat by baking the herbs in an oven to get the moisture out.

Once dried, herbs can be kept in paper bags or stuffed into plastic bags. You can also use glass jars with lids.

Light, heat and oxygen are the enemies of herb potency, so store your herbs in a cool, dark place, like a cellar or cupboard far from any heat source. To minimize the oxygen around stored herbs, fill your containers as full as possible and move the herbs to smaller containers as you use them.

Using Medicinal Herbs

There are many easy ways to use medicinal herbs. Whether you use them as foods, introduce them as seasonings or make teas, you'll get the benefit of their healing properties.

I have nothing against taking vitamin and mineral supplements. In fact, I suggest them for many of the conditions discussed in this book. But an ounce of fruit or vegetables has many more useful constituents than a pound of purified supplements.

My favorite way to use herbs is simply as foods or mixed into foods. In the United States, we make a distinction between foods and drugs, but in many cases there is no real difference. Is garlic, for example, a food or a drug? The correct answer is that it's both. The same goes for all of the culinary spices and many of the herbs discussed throughout this book.

Making Meals That Heal

When it comes to meals that heal, I think it's hard to beat a big mixed green salad, a bowl of vegetable soup (minestrone, which I often call Medistrone) and a fruit salad topped with some herbs such as mint, basil or cinnamon.

In the early 1990s, I was involved with the Designer Food Program of the National Institutes of Health (NIH). The idea was to identify medicinal chemicals, such as plant estrogens (phytoestrogens), which appear to reduce the risk of breast cancer, in plants and to breed or augment these chemicals in food plants.

While the people I worked with in the Designer Food Program were all very bright, charming and well-intentioned, we had some differences of opinion. They wanted to pump plant chemicals (phytochemicals) into foods, while I kept saying that the beneficial chemicals were already there—if you knew where to look. For example, phytoestrogens abound in most beans. If you want to take a big step toward preventing breast cancer, eat bean soup or a bean salad a few times a week, try some Mexican food with refried beans or add tofu to just about anything.

The More Servings, the Better

Many of those in the Designer Food Program endorsed the Strive for Five program promoted by the NIH to encourage Americans to eat five servings a day of fruits and vegetables. An enormous amount of research shows that as fruit and vegetable consumption increases, risk of all the major cancers decreases. In fact, the risk of heart disease, diabetes and many other diseases declines as well. Based on this research, the NIH figured that it was prudent to recommend *at least* five servings a day of fruit and vegetables.

Unfortunately, few Americans get their five a day. And even that goal is short-sighted, in my opinion. I personally think people should strive for at least ten a day—five fruits and five veggies, seasoned with five different herbs and garnished with five different nuts.

As Hippocrates supposedly said, "Let your food be your medicine." Amen to that, especially if you add lots of medicinal spices.

To encourage as many servings of healing foods as possible, I've scattered several recipes throughout this book. But I would certainly never pretend to be a great cook: I rarely measure ingredients at home, and I almost never cook the same dish exactly the same way. I go with a little of this and a handful of that, trusting my taste buds and the wisdom of using as broad a range of fruits, vegetables and herbs as possible. My "recipes" may seem imprecise at times, but the objective is to get you to experiment as much as possible with these tasty herbs. What pleases your palate may not please mine, and vice versa.

How to Make a Healing Tea

You can make a good tea with dried herbs. You can even pop open capsules of powdered herbs and use the contents to make tea. But whenever possible, I use fresh herbs, at least in spring, summer and fall.

Why? Simply because fresh herbs are more fun and more flavorful.

The main difference between fresh herbs and dried herbs is their water content. Leaf for leaf, herbs retain their supply of medicinal phytochemicals even after they've been dried for a while. But phytochemicals are more concentrated in dried herbs because they contain less water. While fresh herbs are about 80 percent water, dried are only about 20 percent. So ounce for ounce, the dried herb is more potent, and when you add it to water, more of the phytochemicals are infused in the tea.

Herbal tea recipes usually assume that you're starting with dried herb material. If you have fresh herbs on hand, you'll need to use four times as much as the recipe calls for if you want to get the same potency.

To Infuse or Decoct?

There are really two types of teas—infusions and decoctions. An infusion is similar to what most people think of as tea. But there's a big difference between beverage teas and medicinal herb infusions. With a beverage tea, you might dunk a tea bag in hot water a few times and then drink it. If you're preparing an herb infusion, the tea should steep for 10 to 20 minutes to allow the therapeutic phytochemicals to pass out of the herb and into the water.

To make a good cup of medicinal tea, here's a good rule of thumb. Start with boiling water and steep your medicinal herbs until the water is cool. If you like to drink it hot, reheat the tea gently.

Decoctions, on the other hand, involve putting herbal material in the water, then boiling or simmering for 10 to 20 minutes. Infusions work best for leaf and flower material because they usually yield their phytochemicals more easily. The decoction method, on the other hand, is typically used for root and twig material because it can be difficult to extract medicinal phytochemicals from them.

Throughout this book, I include suggestions for amounts of herbs to be used in infusions and decoctions. But I must confess that I make my own herb teas the same way I cook—a little of this, a handful of that. In summer I cruise my garden, grabbing whichever aromatic herbs I pass—sometimes more than a dozen—taking bigger portions of the delicate-smelling herbs and smaller portions of the coarse-scented herbs like dittany, horsebalm and thyme. Like my soups and salads, no two of my herb teas are exactly the same.

Suggestions and Safety

What I'm leading up to is this: Use the suggestions in this book as just that— suggestions. I've concentrated mostly on herbs that are safe even in amounts considerably greater than those suggested in the recipes, so don't feel concerned if you use a bit more or less than the recipe suggests. (When exact dosages are extremely important, I note that. And whenever any precautions are needed, I note that as well.)

If there is no recipe for a specific herb, try making an infusion or decoction with one to two teaspoons of plant material. Then tinker with the amounts to suit your personal needs. You can't expect all medicinal teas to taste good; some of them are quite bitter. But if you like the taste and want a stronger tea, it's okay to use a little more of the herb next time around. I mask unpleasant tastes with powdered or real lemonade. The acidity may even extract more of certain medicinal chemicals.

At the same time, however, you must remember that these herbs are medicine. You have to pay attention to how your body responds to the herb and adjust your dose accordingly. If you're looking to relax and end up feeling overly sedated, for example, you'll want to make a weaker tea the next time you're using that particular herb. Our personal chemistries may be just as variable as the herbs'.

As for frequency, I typically suggest one to three cups of tea a day. Again, these are merely suggestions. In general, I wouldn't recommend much more than four cups of most herbal teas per day.

Tinctures and Vinegars

Classically, a tincture is made by steeping herb material in drinkable alcohol, such as ethyl alcohol (ethanol). My personal favorite when I'm creating my own tinctures is cheap vodka. It works just fine.

The alcohol extracts a great deal of the medicinal essence of the herb. Tinctures have longer shelf lives than dried herbs or capsules.

You can buy ready-made tinctures at most places that sell herbs. You can also make your own quite easily.

To make a tincture, you can use anything from 40-proof alcohol to almost 200-proof, which translates as anything from 20 percent alcohol to almost pure alcohol. Most herbalists suggest two ounces of dried herb (or a loose handful of fresh herb) per pint of alcohol. Allow your herb-alcohol mixture to stand for about a week, shaking it occasionally. Then strain it. Discard the plant material (preferably in the compost pile) and store the tincture in a bottle with a dropper lid.

Tincture dosages can run anywhere from 5 to 50 drops or from a fraction of a dropperful to several dropperfuls. Sometimes they're even measured in teaspoons or tablespoons. I usually add tinctures to beverage herbal teas or to juices.

One advantage of buying a tincture is that appropriate dosages are generally indicated on the label.

While alcohol is a great preservative, we want to pickle the herb, not the consumer. One nonalcoholic option that's often available these days is glycerides, tinctures that have been prepared using glycerin rather than alcohol. These are nice options for infants or for recovering alcoholics who wish to avoid alcohol in any form.

Herbal vinegars are another good option, and you can even make your own. To do this, simply steep your herbs in vinegar rather than alcohol. The same ratios might be used: one pint of vinegar for every one to two ounces of dried herb or loose handful of fresh herb.

You can use many herbal vinegars straight as salad dressings, which can be especially helpful for people who are overweight. Herbal vinegars can also be added to soups or cooked vegetables.

Using Poultices and Compresses

A poultice is a wad of chopped, fresh (or dried but remoistened) plant material that is applied directly to a wound or infection on the skin and usually held in place by a wet dressing that is covered by a bandage.

It's best to soften the herb first to coax out more of the medicinal phytochemicals. You can do this by boiling, steaming, chewing or pounding it. Then shape the material into a small, coin-size wad that can lie flat against the wound. Many herbalists recommend mixing one part herb with three parts water, alcohol or vinegar thickened with flour to make the poultice easier to handle and apply. In a pinch, you can simply ball up some whole leaf and use that.

Poultices work primarily at the application site, typically preventing infection and hastening the healing of wounds. But there are doubtless many compounds in poultice plants that pass through the skin and have internal benefits as well.

Compresses are clean cloths that have been dipped in an herbal solution—an infusion, decoction, tincture or vinegar. Compresses can be used in two ways. You might hold a poultice in place with a compress, in which case it doubles as a bandage. Or you might apply it directly to the skin. This type of compress is also known as a fomentation.

Soothing Salves

Many commercial salves contain herbs, and probably your best bet is to buy a salve rather than make it. Making your own salves is a pretty messy business, but you can certainly go that route if you choose. Making salves involves mixing medicinal herbs with water, beeswax, animal fat (lard or lanolin), vegetable fat (corn oil, Crisco, margarine or olive or safflower oil) and other ingredients to create spreadable lotions.

I confess that I've never had much luck mixing up salves. Mine tend to be either too runny or too dry. But other herbalists are much better at it.

If you'd like to try making a salve, start with pulverized herb and cover it with water. Boil or simmer for 15 to 30 minutes, then let it cool. Add some oil, then gently heat the oily mixture until the water has evaporated, perhaps 15 to 30 minutes.

Finally, add beeswax and/or a fat to give your salve the proper consistency. Cool before using. A well-prepared salve can keep for up to a year. Salves can be used like poultices, except that you often don't need the bandage.

If you'd rather not make salves from scratch, you can also simply add pulverized, simmered herb material to any of the commercial skin ointments sold in drugstores.

Healing with Aromatherapy

Aromatherapy is the treatment of medical conditions with the aromatic essential oils of fragrant herbs. Aromatherapists often use essential oils from the mint family, which includes such aromatherapeutic superstars as lavender (a tranquilizer) and rosemary (a stimulant).

The essential oils used in aromatherapy, which come in little vials, are extremely concentrated. You can simply sniff directly from the vial, or you can use the oil for massage.

Since the oils are so concentrated, they can be irritating to the skin. If you're using an oil for massage, first dilute it by adding a few drops to vegetable oil or massage lotion. If you doubt that essential oils can pass through your skin, here's an experiment for you to try: Massage a few drops of diluted lavender oil into your skin. Within a short time, your friends may notice that you have lavender breath when you exhale.

Another nice way to use essential oils is to add a few drops to your bath. (You can also use a handful of fresh or dried herbs if you choose.) Since many of the fragrant compounds are readily absorbed through the skin, this is a particularly pleasant way to get your medicine. If you have insomnia, for example, I suggest adding sedative lavender and lemon balm (also known as melissa) to your bath. I bet you'll fall asleep more easily and sleep more soundly.

Whatever you do, though, do not ingest essential oils. Many are quite toxic, and as little as a half-teaspoon can kill you. (A few essential oils can be taken in diluted form, but this is not something that you can experiment with on your own. An experienced herbal practitioner may occasionally recommend ingesting diluted essential oils.)

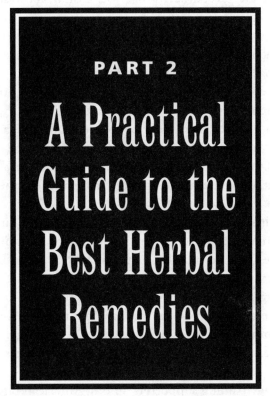

PART 2

A Practical
Guide to the
Best Herbal
Remedies

Aging

Being a botanist, I have a particular interest in herbs that can hold back the aging process. But I'm forced to admit that lifestyle changes—such as eating healthfully, exercising regularly, and not smoking or drinking—are a whole lot more important than herbs in helping you stay youthful. These changes should form the foundation of any anti-aging herbal treatments that you decide to try.

That said, there are several herbs that you should know about for holding back the ravages of age.

★★★ **Put ginkgo at the top of your list.** This is the most intriguing herb for counteracting the neurological slings and arrows of aging. There's good European research showing that it helps improve blood flow to the brain. Some studies suggest that ginkgo helps people with Alzheimer's disease and other forms of dementia become more alert and sociable, think more clearly, feel better and remember more. In Europe, many older people regularly take a standardized extract of this herb to help keep them mentally fit.

You can try 60 to 240 milligrams of standardized extracts a day, but don't go any higher than that. In large amounts, ginkgo may cause diarrhea, irritability and restlessness.

★★ **Discover ginseng's anti-aging effects.** The Chinese and Koreans revere ginseng as the Fountain of Youth. They regard this herb as a tonic for the elderly because it tones the skin and muscles, helps improve appetite and digestion and restores depleted sexual energy.

While on a trip to China in 1978 for the express purpose of investigating ginseng, I had one elderly Chinese man tell me not to waste this herb on young people. He said I should save it for old age, when it would make me feel young again. I'm almost ready. The house is paid off, and I have five species of ginseng growing on my six-acre farmette.

Ginseng is slowly gaining supporters among American physicians. One big booster is Andrew Weil, M.D., herb advocate, professor at the University of Arizona College of Medicine in Tucson and author of *Natural Health, Natural Medicine*. He frequently recommends ginseng to help strengthen people who are weakened by old age or chronic illness.

★★ **Pick evening primrose.** The seeds of this lovely night-flowering blossom contain an oil rich in gamma-linolenic acid (GLA), a substance that has excited a great deal of research interest in the past few years. GLA seems to help alleviate several conditions: premenstrual syndrome (PMS); eczema, a chronic skin condition that causes itchy, red, scaly patches; diabetic polyneuropathy, a type of nerve damage associated with diabetes; and perhaps even alcoholism and obesity. It also shows promise against America's biggest killers, heart disease and cancer.

Allergies

Allergies are abnormal reactions to everyday substances. They are caused by the immune system's overreaction to histamine, a chemical that the body releases to fight microbial invaders. But in allergies, the invaders are not viruses or bacteria. They are harmless substances: pollens, dust, mold spores or harmless microscopic bugs called dust mites that live in carpets, clothing and bedding.

Standard medical treatment for allergies involves taking decongestants and antihistamines. Decongestants open clogged nasal passages and have drying action. Antihistamines suppress the body's release of histamine. In severe cases, doctors prescribe immunotherapy, popularly known as allergy shots.

You won't be surprised to learn that I prefer "greener," more natural approaches for dealing with allergy symptoms. Here are some helpful herbs.

★★ **Snuff out symptoms with garlic.** These may be beneficial because of the high concentrations of compounds such as quercetin found in these plants. These compounds retard inflammatory reactions. If you have allergies, I'd suggest adding generous amounts of these foods to your menu.

★★ **Go on the offensive with ginkgo.** The leaf extract of the stately ginkgo tree contains several unique substances (ginkgolides) that interfere with the action of a chemical that the body produces—platelet-activating factor, or PAF. PAF plays a key role in triggering allergies, asthma and inflammation. My own allergies have never been severe enough to make me reach for ginkgo, but if they got bad, I would probably try it. You can try 60 to 240 milligrams of standardized extract a day, but don't go any higher than that. In large amounts, ginkgo may cause diarrhea, irritability and restlessness.

★★ **Take the sting out of allergies with stinging nettle.** Some good research shows that nettle preparations may effectively treat allergic nasal symptoms. Every spring, visitors to my herb garden dig up roots from my nettle patch to treat their hay fever. We shouldn't be surprised that nettle does, in fact, help relieve allergy symptoms. For centuries, cultures around the world have used this herb to treat nasal and respiratory troubles: coughs, runny nose, chest congestion, asthma, whooping cough and even tuberculosis. At a Columbia University Workshop on Botanical Medicine for Physicians, herb advocate Andrew Weil, M.D., professor at the University of Arizona College of Medicine in

Tucson and author of *Natural Health, Natural Medicine*, said that he knew of nothing so dramatic as the allergy (hay fever) relief afforded by freeze-dried nettle leaves.

Amenorrhea

Herbs that bring on menstrual flow—for whatever reason—are known as emmenagogues. Back in the days before modern medicine, women often used emmenagogues for two reasons. Some used the herbs as a kind of morning-after contraception, because not much else was available. Others used them to treat amenorrhea—the medical term for lack of menstruation in women who should be having regular periods. Emmenagogues are no longer necessary for contraception, but they might still help with amenorrhea.

You should see your doctor for a diagnosis if you have amenorrhea. The standard medical treatment is hormone therapy, but hormone treatments are tricky, require sophisticated monitoring and in many cases, fail to get results. In my experience, emmenagogues often restore normal menstrual flow and provide considerable emotional relief. You might ask your doctor about trying these safe and gentle herbs before resorting to hormones.

From the longer list in my database, here are some of my favorites.

★★★ **Jump-start your periods with chasteberry.** In one small study, 20 women with amenorrhea were given 40 drops daily of a chasteberry extract, then were monitored for six months. Fifteen completed the study, and 10 of them had their menstrual cycles restored.

Amenorrhea is often associated with elevated blood levels of the hormone prolactin, and drugs that reduce prolactin usually restore the menstrual cycle to normal. Chasteberry acts just like these drugs.

The typical dose is 20 milligrams per day of a tincture made from the fruits. In Germany, herbal medicines are widely used and often recommended by doctors. One popular German amenorrhea preparation (Femisana) is a tincture of chasteberry fruits, along with greater celandine, black cohosh and pasque-flower.

★★ **Get back on track with black cohosh and blue cohosh.** These were the American Indians' two favorite herbs for gynecological complaints. It turns out that black cohosh has potent estrogen-like activity, and blue cohosh stimulates uterine contractions.

★ **Drink dill tea.** The compound apiole in dill is such a powerful emmenagogue that most herbalists I respect warn pregnant women not to use it in medicinal concentrations. (Don't panic, though—eating a dill pickle is okay.) If you want to encourage menstrual flow, you can brew a tea using two teaspoons of mashed seeds.

Arthritis

Arthritis literally means "joint inflammation." There are more than 100 different diseases that produce joint pain and inflammation. But when people say "arthritis," they usually mean osteoarthritis.

Also known as degenerative joint disease, osteoarthritis is the most prevalent of more than a dozen different kinds of arthritis. The hips, knees, spine and the tiny joints of the hands and feet are most frequently affected. Osteoarthritis usually develops gradually, beginning with minor aches that eventually lead to extended pain, stiffness, swelling and limited range of motion. Symptoms sometimes subside with gentle physical activity, but not always.

Another common form of arthritis is the rheumatoid variety. Rheumatoid arthritis (RA) has a nasty reputation because it can cause crippling joint deformity. But many Americans with RA have milder, noncrippling cases that flare up and subside mysteriously.

Frequently, both hands are affected, but RA can strike other joints as well. In addition to joint pain, swelling and warmth, possible symptoms include fatigue, fever, loss of appetite, enlarged lymph nodes, lumps under the skin and muscle stiffness after sleep or inactivity. Stiffness usually subsides with moderate activity.

Fortunately, there are a number of other herbs that can help.

★★★ **Treat your joints to ginger and turmeric.** In one study, Indian researchers gave three to seven grams (1½ to 3½ teaspoons) of ginger a day to 18 people with osteoarthritis and 28 with rheumatoid arthritis. More than 75 percent of those participating in the study reported at least some relief from pain and swelling. Even after more than two years of taking these high doses of ginger, none of the people reported side effects.

The curcumin in turmeric is a close chemical relative of some compounds found in ginger, so I'm not surprised that this herb also has a major reputation as an arthritis treatment.

You can enjoy both herbs in a wide variety of spicy dishes as well as use them to make teas.

★★★ **Promote relief with pineapple.** Some intriguing research suggests that bromelain, a chemical in pineapple, helps prevent inflammation. I think it's also a good bet for people with arthritis. Bromelain can help the body get rid of immune antigen complex, compounds that are implicated in some arthritic conditions. It also helps digest fibrin, another compound suspected of being involved in some types of arthritis. If you need an excuse to indulge yourself with fresh, ripe pineapple, this is it.

★★★ **Apply red pepper cream.** Red pepper causes some pain on the tongue, but ironically, it interferes with pain perception elsewhere around the body. The pain-relieving chemical in red pepper, capsaicin, triggers the body to release endorphins, nature's own opiates. Red pepper also contains aspirin-like compounds known as salicylates.

You can make a tea by mixing red pepper into water, but it would be a whole lot more pleasurable to have your red pepper cooked in a variety of spicy dishes. For a quick hit, try a splash of hot-pepper sauce in tomato juice.

Compounds in red pepper can also help relieve arthritis when you apply the herb to the skin. Researchers have discovered that you'll get significant pain relief if you apply capsaicin cream directly to painful arthritic joints four times daily. In one study of this treatment, the capsaicin cream reduced RA pain by more than half. Osteoarthritis pain was reduced by about one-third.

Capsaicin creams are generally believed safe and effective for arthritis. Look for capsaicin in the ingredient list of over-the-counter pain creams such as Zostrix or Capzasin-P or ask your doctor for a prescription capsaicin product. If you use a capsaicin cream, be sure to wash your hands thoroughly afterward: You don't want to get it in your eyes. Also, since some people are quite sensitive to this compound, you should test it on a small area of skin to make sure that it's okay for you to use before using it on a larger area. If it seems to irritate your skin, discontinue use.

Asthma

Asthma is a chronic respiratory ailment that causes wheezing, coughing, chest congestion, shortness of breath and often tremendous anxiety about being unable to breathe. Doctors treat asthma with a variety of drugs—among them, theophylline (Aerolate, Theo-Dur)—that open up the bronchial tubes. These drugs, known as bronchodilators, are often taken with an inhaler.

If I had asthma, I'd certainly follow a physician's recommendations. This is a potentially fatal illness. But for my treatment, if my doctor suggested theophylline, I'd prefer to get it from its many natural sources, chief among them the plants containing caffeine.

★★★ **Get a kick from caffeine.** Coffee, tea, caffeinated colas and cocoa, as well as chocolate candy, are derived from plants and count as herbal products. And all contain caffeine as well as other compounds that may help fend off asthma.

Actually, coffee, tea, caffeinated cola drinks, cocoa and chocolate have more than caffeine. All reportedly contain two other major natural anti-asthmatic compounds, theobromine and theophylline, which, along with caffeine, belong to a family of chemicals called xanthines. These chemicals help stop bronchospasms and open constricted bronchial passages.

Levels of these anti-asthmatic compounds vary, depending on the strength of the brew and other factors. But in general, a cup of coffee has the highest levels (about 100 milligrams of caffeine per cup), while a cup of tea or cocoa or a 12-ounce can of cola has about half that amount. A 1½-ounce chocolate bar has a little less than a can of cola.

★★★ **Breathe better with stinging nettle.** Four hundred years ago, the British herbalist Nicholas Culpeper claimed that nettle roots or leaves, used in juice or tea, were "safe and sure medicines to open the pipes and passages of the lungs."

For many years, Australians have viewed nettle as a good treatment for asthma. Aussies drink the juice of the roots and leaves mixed with honey or sugar, and they firmly believe that it relieves bronchial troubles. But Americans didn't catch on until a few years ago, when a scientific study was published showing that nettle is a potent antihistamine. Now nettle is increasingly recommended for hay fever and asthma. Friends with allergies and asthma visit my garden regularly to dig up my nettle patch. (You'll need to wear gloves when harvesting stinging nettle leaves, but the stinging hairs lose their sting when the leaves are cooked.)

★★ **Make anise and fennel your allies.** The Greeks use teas made from these herbs for asthma and other respiratory ailments. They both contain helpful chemicals—creosol and alpha-pinene—that help loosen bronchial secretions. Fennel seeds (actually fruits) can contain as much as 8,800 parts per million (ppm) of alpha-pinene. Ironically, despite its traditional use for respiratory problems, anise is no superstar. It has only 360 ppm of alpha-pinene.

Athlete's Foot

Athlete's foot, medically known as tinea pedis, is a superficial fungal infection. Athlete's foot fungus needs moisture and darkness to grow. That's why both conventional doctors and alternative practitioners recommend keeping the feet dry. And of course, your feet are drier if you go around barefoot rather than keeping your toes all trapped and humid in dark, closed shoes.

Here are the herbs I recommend for athlete's foot.

★★★ **Get rid of fungus with garlic.** This is my first-choice treatment. It's one of the most widely recommended antifungal antiseptics, and for good reason. Many scientifically rigorous studies show that it's effective in treating athlete's foot and other fungal infections, notably vaginal yeast infections.

A garlic footbath might be malodorous, but it usually relieves itching and burning between the toes. I suggest putting several crushed garlic cloves in a basin with warm water and a little rubbing alcohol.

★★★ **Be generous with ginger.** According to my database, ginger ranks second among all herbs in the number of antifungal compounds with a total of 23. One compound—caprylic acid—is so potent that a chemist I know suggests taking three capsules a day for all manner of fungal infections. Of course, unless you're a chemist, you probably can't get pure caprylic acid, which is why I recommend using ginger instead.

You can prepare a strong decoction by adding an ounce of chopped ginger root to a cup of boiling water. Simmer for 20 minutes and apply it directly to the problem areas twice a day with a cotton ball or clean cloth.

★★★ **Dab on teatree oil.** Teatree oil is a powerful antiseptic that's very useful against athlete's foot. Dilute the oil with an equal amount of water or vegetable oil and apply it directly to the affected area three times a day using a cotton ball or clean cloth. Just don't ingest it. Like so many other essential plant oils, small amounts of teatree oil, on the order of a few teaspoons, can be fatal.

Backache

It seems that everywhere I look, people have back problems. That's not surprising, because aching backs are one of America's most prevalent health problems. Estimates vary, but the experts generally agree that somewhere between two and five million Americans suffer serious back pain each year.

Immediately after a back injury or a flare-up of back pain, doctors recommend pain-relieving and anti-inflammatory medications such as aspirin and other nonsteroidal anti-inflammatory drugs. For really bad pain, stronger medications might be necessary, including codeine or other narcotics. If you're in serious pain, I'd suggest taking whatever the doctor orders.

For lesser pain or lingering pain, there are a number of herbal alternatives that can prove helpful.

★★★ **Chase pain with red pepper.** Red pepper contains a marvelous pain-relieving chemical—capsaicin—that is so potent that a tiny amount provides the active ingredient in some powerful pharmaceutical topical analgesics. One product, Zostrix, contains only 0.025 percent capsaicin.

At this point, I don't know (or care) whether red pepper's effectiveness is due to capsaicin's ability to interfere with pain perception, to its ability to trigger release of the body's own pain-relieving endorphins, to its salicylates, or to all three. All I know is that it works.

When you use capsaicin cream, be sure to wash your hands thoroughly afterward: You don't want to get it in your eyes. Also, since some people are quite sensitive to this compound, you should test it on a small area of skin to make sure that it's okay before using it on a larger area. If it seems to irritate your skin, discontinue use.

★★★ **Discover herbal aspirin.** I have no problem with taking aspirin, since it was originally derived from an herbal source. It originally came from compounds known as salicylates that occur naturally in willow bark, meadowsweet and wintergreen. Any of these herbs can be made into pain-relieving teas.

Many salicylate-rich plants also contain methyl-salicylate, an aspirin-like compound with a particularly pleasing smell. One is wintergreen. Another is birch bark, once used by American Indians to make a tea that they drank or applied externally to treat lower back pain. On occasion I have made such teas by throwing roughly a handful of birch bark or wintergreen into a cup or two of boiling water and letting it steep for about ten minutes. (Remember, though, that if you're allergic to aspirin, you probably shouldn't use aspirin-like herbs, either.)

★★ **Relax muscles with mint.** You will find the compounds menthol and camphor in many over-the-counter backache medications. They are chemicals that can help ease the muscle tightness that contributes to many bad backs. Menthol is a natural constituent of plants in the mint family, particularly peppermint and spearmint, although the aromatic oils of all the other mints contain it as well. Camphor occurs in spike lavender, hyssop and coriander.

Bad Breath

Most bad breath is caused by bacteria in the mouth. Bacteria produce wastes that smell, well, bad. During the day, oxygen-rich saliva acts as a natural mouthwash, keeping oral bacteria largely at bay. But at night, salivation slows, and the chemical environment of the mouth shifts from mildly acidic to mildly alkaline, which encourages the growth of odor-causing bacteria. By morning, you have what those commercials call "morning mouth."

In at least one-third of people with halitosis, the cause is gum (periodontal) disease. Bacteria worm their way down into the gums below the tooth line, where not even the fanciest toothbrush can reach. As they grow, they destroy gum tissue. If not treated, this gum damage eventually causes tooth loss. At the same time, the bacteria release the wastes that cause bad breath.

Flossing can help control gum disease. So can a mouthwash containing the right herbs. But chronic halitosis may also be a sign of several other conditions, according to Israel Kleinberg, M.D., chairman of the Department of Oral Biology and Pathology at the State University of New York at Stony Brook. Some are quite serious: cirrhosis of the liver, diabetes, kidney failure and cancer in the upper respiratory tract, among others. If your bad breath just won't quit, it's a good idea to discuss it with your doctor.

Most bad breath is just a passing inconvenience, and there are a number of herbs that can help erase it.

★★★ **Clear the air with cardamom.** In my database, cardamom is the richest source of the compound cineole, a potent antiseptic that also kills bad breath bacteria. And it may have more than just a breath-freshening benefit if you use it during a romantic date. Arab cultures consider it an aphrodisiac. Try chewing cardamom fruits (seeds). I chew them for a while and then spit them out. I also add them to herbal teas and liqueurs.

★★★ **End odor with eucalyptus.** Many commercial mouthwashes contain alcohol, which helps kill odor-causing bacteria, and eucalyptol, a compound that is derived from eucalyptus oil and is rich in cineole.

Many other herbs are also rich in cineole. While none of them except cardamom come close to eucalyptus's cineole content, any of these herbs would help freshen the breath: spearmint, rosemary, sweet Annie, ginger, nutmeg, lavender, bee balm, peppermint, tansy, yarrow, cinnamon, basil, turmeric, lemon leaf, hyssop, tarragon, lemon verbena or fennel.

★★★ **Nibble on parsley.** My cousin Suzie, who has high blood pressure, called recently to ask what I might recommend. I advised her to take garlic to lower her blood pressure, plus parsley to minimize the halitosis caused by the garlic. Bright green parsley is a rich source of the green plant pigment, chlorophyll, which is a powerful breath freshener. Munch some parsley after meals, after drinking coffee or after eating or drinking anything that might cause malodorous breath.

In fact, it's a good idea to refrigerate fresh sprigs of parsley and other plants rich in chlorophyll, notably basil and cilantro, and nibble as needed.

Bladder Infections

You're probably going to want to know right off the bat whether cranberry juice really helps prevent bladder infections. This one is easy: Yes, there is reason to believe that it does. And there are several other herbal treatments that can help as well.

Bladder infection, also called cystitis and urinary tract infection (UTI), is a bacterial infection that causes painful urination and a feeling that the bladder never completely empties. It can also cause fever and low back pain. Urine from an infected bladder may smell strong and contain tinges of blood. (If you develop any of these symptoms, you should see your doctor for treatment.)

Some 80 percent of bladder infections are caused by bacteria from the anal area, notably *Escherichia coli*, a microorganism that lives in the digestive tract.

Doctors treat UTIs with antibiotics. But quite often, natural approaches—foods and herbs—work just as well.

★★★ **Treat your bladder with berries.** I'm enthusiastic about blueberries and cranberries. Folk practitioners have claimed for a long time that they help. A study published in the *Journal of the American Medical Association* showed that certain compounds in cranberry and blueberry juice prevent bacteria from adhering to the bladder walls. And if they can't stick to the bladder walls, they won't cause infection there.

The only problem with the cranberry juice prescription is that you have to drink a lot of it. Naturopaths suggest drinking 17 ounces a day to treat UTIs. The juice is naturally tart and must be sweetened to be palatable, meaning that this prescription is rather high in calories. If you try this, make sure you adjust the rest of your diet accordingly.

★★★ **To prevent infections, eat yogurt.** While this isn't an herb, I won't hold that against it. It's too good a natural healer to exclude from this chapter. Studies show that the active bacterial cultures in yogurt help prevent both bladder infections and yeast infections. The trick, of course, is to eat yogurt with live cultures. If it has live cultures, the label will say so.

How about yogurt with blueberries and cranberry juice for an infection-fighting breakfast?

★★ **Drink parsley juice.** After cranberry and blueberry, juices that are often recommended for bladder infections include carrot, celery, cucumber and parsley. Parsley in particular has a long history of use for bladder problems, and no wonder. Good research shows that it's a diuretic that helps empty the bladder.

Body Odor

The chemistry of armpits is rather interesting. Much of our body odor comes from emanations of the apocrine sweat glands, most of which are located in the underarm area. If we don't wash it off regularly—every six hours or so—bacteria begin to colonize these apocrine secretions. And a while later we develop . . . guess what?

In addition to poor hygiene, body odor may be caused by a zinc deficiency, diabetes or liver disease, chronic constipation and certain parasites. Vegetarians claim that meat-eaters have more body odor.

Bathing is probably the best way to control body odor, but if you don't feel socially at ease without a deodorant, there's no need to use commercial roll-ons or sprays.

Herbs have a long and illustrious history of use as deodorants. Not surprisingly, the herbs most widely used all have antibacterial action against the microorganisms that make our apocrine secretions smell unpleasant. Here are some to try.

★★★ **Banish BO with coriander and licorice.** My trusty database shows that coriander and licorice both contain 20 chemicals with antibacterial action. Oregano and rosemary have 19; ginger, 17; nutmeg, 15; cinnamon and cumin, 11; and bay, 10.

Looking at the quantity of bactericidal compounds in various herbs—as opposed to the number of compounds—we find that licorice contains up to 33 percent bactericidal compounds.

All of the herbs mentioned so far should have some impact against the bacteria that cause body odor. One way to use these deodorant herbs is to powder them and rub them into your underarms. It's an effective approach, but it might also stain clothing. So instead, I would suggest making a strong tea of the herb or herbs of your choice, soaking a cloth in it and applying the moist cloth as a compress for a few minutes.

Add plenty of sage, and if various reasonably well-informed sources are correct, your tea might also provide antiperspirant benefit.

★ **Dry out with baking soda and cornstarch.** Apply a mixture of these powders in malodorous areas. The drying action of both powders helps, and as anyone who has ever used an open box of baking soda to control odors in the refrigerator knows, baking soda has deodorant action. I know that baking soda is not an herb, but it's such a natural approach to this problem that I thought I'd include it.

Bronchitis

I'm not personally acquainted with the TV newsman Walter Cronkite, but he and I have something in common. Over a decade ago, on independent trips to China, our hosts gave both of us honeysuckle tea. I was given the tea for flu. He got the tea for bronchitis, the inflammation of the bronchial tubes that causes persistent cough, chest congestion and often the production of a lot of thick, sticky phlegm.

Both of us recovered quickly, and I'm inclined to believe that this ancient herbal remedy helped. Doctors tend to scoff at such statements. Our two case studies are merely what the scientists often dismiss as anecdotal evidence.

All right, so our cases don't really prove anything. But there's more to honeysuckle—and other herbs—than just anecdotes. And these days, there are a lot of scientific studies to back that up.

Bronchitis has several possible causes. It may be bacterial or viral, or it may be caused by some chronic irritant such as cigarette smoking or exposure to certain chemicals. Sometimes the germs and irritants work together: A smoker catches a cold and the cough turns into bronchitis.

Bronchitis may clear up by itself without any treatment, but it can also linger and sometimes become chronic. That's why I favor treating it. Here are some of my favorite natural bronchitis remedies.

★★ **Use eucalyptus to clear your lungs.** Eucalyptus oil is a good expectorant (a substance that helps loosen phlegm). Commission E, the body of natural medicine experts that makes herbal recommendations to Germany's health advisers, has endorsed inhaling eucalyptus vapors to treat bronchitis and coughs.

Taken internally, eucalyptus leaf tea might have the same benefits. I say this because, after you ingest eucalyptus and your body absorbs it, part of its essential oil is secreted through your lungs. So you get the antiseptic, cooling and expectorant properties of eucalyptus right where you need them.

★★ **Beat bronchitis with garlic.** Eating a lot of garlic can help prevent bronchitis because garlic is filled with chemicals that are antiviral and antibacterial.

Garlic may also protect you from colds and flu because "garlic breath" keeps people from getting too close to you. (Just joking!) Actually, there is a serious side to garlic breath that serves to demonstrate just how useful this herb is in treating respiratory complaints. In the body, garlic releases aromatic chemicals, including allicin, one of the most potent broad-spectrum plant antiseptics. These aromatic compounds are excreted through the lungs—hence garlic breath. The presence of these compounds in the lungs is good. It means that, as with eucalyptus, you get garlic's active constituents right where you need them.

To minimize garlic breath, you can chew on a few sprigs of parsley.

★★ **Mull over mullein.** Mullein has been endorsed by Commission E for respiratory complaints because it has expectorant properties. It can help bring up that sticky phlegm. In fact, mullein has been an herbal favorite for respiratory ailments for thousands of years. In addition to its expectorant action, it soothes the throat, has bactericidal activity and helps stop the muscle spasms that trigger coughs.

Bruises

Those black-and-blue marks known as bruises are actually caused by blood that leaks out of capillaries just under the skin, usually after an injury. Black eyes are more common in men than women, while blue spots occur most frequently on the legs of older women.

Many experts, naturopaths in particular, recommend bromelain—a protein-digesting enzyme in pineapple—as a treatment for bruises. I'm not that strongly in favor of bromelain, however. In fact, I don't think pineapple and bromelain represent the best natural approach to either the prevention or treatment of bruises.

Perhaps it is as effective as the naturopaths say, but personally I'd suggest fruits that are rich in vitamin C and bioflavonoids, such as oranges and other citrus fruits. Bioflavonoids are beneficial nutrients that often show up in foods that are rich in vitamin C, and together these nutrients help strengthen capillary walls, making them more resistant to the blood leakage that causes bruises. When bruises occur, vitamin C and bioflavonoids help capillary walls—and black-and-blue marks—heal more rapidly.

While you're feasting on pineapple and citrus fruit, you might also try some other traditional herbal treatments that have scientific merit.

★ **End inflammation with arnica.** This herb, also known as mountain daisy, is helpful in treating bruises, according to Commission E, the body of experts that advises the German government about herbs.

Arnica, which has pain-relieving, antiseptic and anti-inflammatory properties, is best reserved for use on the skin. While you should not take it internally to treat bruises, you can make a healing solution using one teaspoon of dried herb per cup of boiling water. Steep until cool and then apply with a clean cloth. Or make the solution using tincture of arnica; a few drops per cup of water will do it. Commercial, mostly homeopathic arnica ointments are also available. Look for a product containing up to 15 percent arnica oil and follow the package directions.

★ **Find comfort in comfrey.** Comfrey is among the oldest herbal remedies for skin problems, dating back to ancient Greece. Modern researchers have discovered that it contains allantoin, a chemical that promotes skin repair. Allantoin is an ingredient in a number of commercial skin creams.

A review of the scientific literature by Commission E uncovered evidence that comfrey is also anti-inflammatory. That's why the commission endorsed applying it to the skin to treat bruises, dislocations and sprains.

To treat bruises, medical anthropologist and herb expert John Heinerman recommends first-aid application of ice packs, then a bandage soaked in comfrey tea. Quick action can prevent some discoloration.

It's probably a good idea not to ingest comfrey, however. It contains pyrrolizidine alkaloids, compounds that are toxic to the liver, and there is some controversy about its safety.

★ **Go ape for grape seeds.** In recent years, a chemical found in grape seeds and pine bark has become a popular, though expensive, supplement. It is sold under the brand name Pycnogenol. According to some naturopaths, Pycnogenol increases levels of vitamin C in the body's cells and strengthens the capillaries against the kind of traumatic injury that causes bruises. I'm not entirely sold on Pycnogenol, but by blending grape seeds into grape juice, you can get some for free.

Burns

Burns come in three degrees of severity. First-degree burns injure only the outermost layer of skin. An ordinary sunburn, for example, is a first-degree burn.

When a burn develops blisters, the injury has penetrated deeper into the skin, and you have a very painful second-degree burn.

The worst type of burn, a third-degree burn, is, oddly, often not painful at all. That's because the injury penetrates so deeply that it destroys the nerves that transmit pain signals to the brain.

Third-degree burns are medical emergencies that always require professional care and typically necessitate hospitalization. And any second-degree burn that covers an area of skin larger than a quarter should receive medical attention.

For first-degree and smaller second-degree burns, there are a number of herbal treatments that can soothe the burn and help bring relief.

★★★ **Allay pain with aloe.** Aloe has been used to treat burns and other wounds since ancient times. But it's not just a folk remedy. Many studies have shown that the gel obtained by slitting open the succulent's fat, leathery leaves relieves burns, including burns caused by radiation treatments for cancer.

My friend Varro Tyler, Ph.D., dean and professor emeritus of pharmacognosy (natural product pharmacy) at Purdue University in West Lafayette, Indiana, cites many studies showing that aloe gel is useful in treating burns, wounds and frostbite.

Scientists are still not certain how aloe speeds the healing of burns, but the herb appears to have several beneficial effects. One study showed that aloe increases the amount of blood flowing to areas of burned tissue, which brings more of the body's healing resources to the area where they're needed.

★ **Soak your skin in lavender.** During the 1920s, French perfume chemist René-Maurice Gattefossé burned his hand in his laboratory. He plunged it into the nearest liquid—a container of lavender oil. The pain subsided quickly and the burn healed with no scarring. This incident may have led to the development of aromatherapy, the use in healing of various essential oils taken from plants.

Other essential oils, such as camomile, camphor, eucalyptus, geranium, onion, peppermint, rosemary and sage, have also been touted as burn treatments. But aromatherapists I know reserve their highest praise for lavender oil. Consider placing a vial on your kitchen windowsill right next to the aloe plant. (Remember, though, that you should never ingest essential oils, as even a small amount can be toxic.)

★ **Discover the soothing properties of plantain.** Plantain is one of the most popular folk herbal remedies for burns in the United States. Juice from the fresh leaves of this plant is applied directly to mild burns. I've used it many times and found it soothing.

Bursitis and Tendinitis

These two disorders are often lumped together, but they're actually two distinct conditions. Bursitis is an inflammation of the bursae, the fluid-filled sacs that help lubricate the joints in places where muscles and tendons meet bone. Tendinitis is an inflammation of the tendons, the tough, elastic, fibrous tissues that connect muscles to bones.

The two terms are often used interchangeably because the bursae are located near tendon-bone connections, and both conditions cause pain in and around the joints. Bursitis and tendinitis also have the same cause—overuse of a particular joint. These kinds of problems show up as a result of sports, as in tennis elbow, and in jobs that require repetitive movement, such as carpentry and butchering. Whatever you call them, though, bursitis and tendinitis really hurt. And interestingly enough, they both respond to the same kinds of treatments.

Physicians generally treat bursitis, tendinitis and related problems with rest and medications that relieve pain and reduce inflammation—aspirin and other nonsteroidal anti-inflammatory drugs and corticosteroids.

I think resting a joint that has been affected by tendinitis or bursitis is a great idea. Ice packs might also help control the pain and inflammation. But don't count on an ice pack to provide complete relief. And while taking aspirin and related drugs is fine, you should be aware that there are also a number of natural alternatives.

★★★ **Try nature's pain relievers.** Willow bark is herbal aspirin. So are meadowsweet and wintergreen. They all contain salicylates, natural precursors of aspirin. To make a tea, I suggest using one to two teaspoons of dried herb per cup of water and boiling it for about 20 minutes. Have a cup two or three times a day. Or try a teaspoon of tincture of any of these herbs three times a day. Remember, though, that if you're allergic to aspirin, you probably shouldn't take aspirin-like herbs, either.

★ **Ease discomfort with echinacea.** This herb, also called coneflower, is good for connective tissue injuries such as tennis elbow, skier's knee and jogger's ankle, according to Michael Moore, author of *Medicinal Plants of the Desert and Canyon West* and one of the nation's leading herbalists. All of these injuries are, in fact, types of tendinitis. He recommends taking up to a half-ounce of echinacea tincture daily until the swelling and pain are reduced. That's a lot of tincture, but echinacea is not hazardous (although it may cause your tongue to tingle or become numb), so it's probably worth a try.

★ **Rely on licorice.** Licorice can be every bit as effective a treatment for bursitis and tendinitis as the commonly prescribed drug hydrocortisone, according to herbal pharmacologist Daniel Mowrey, Ph.D., author of *The Scientific Validation of Herbal Medicine* and *Herbal Tonic Therapies*. Plus, the herb has none of the usual side effects, such as weight gain, indigestion, insomnia and lowered resistance to infection, that are associated with cortisone and hydrocortisone. From what I know of licorice's anti-inflammatory effects, I believe this herb is worth trying. (While licorice and its extracts are safe for normal use in moderate amounts—up to about three cups of tea a day—long-term use or ingestion of larger amounts can produce headache, lethargy, sodium and water retention, excessive loss of potassium and high blood pressure.)

Canker Sores

Canker sores are painful, craterlike ulcers that form in the mouth or on the inner lips. Also known as aphthous ulcers, canker sores usually clear up by themselves within a week or so, but they often recur, sometimes in the form of multiple sores.

Doctors don't have much to offer people with canker sores. They often prescribe antibiotics or corticosteroids, medications that help relieve pain and inflammation. But neither of these treatments helps much. So even doctors tend to recommend traditional relief—ice to alleviate the pain and rinsing the mouth with warm saltwater several times a day.

Doctors also suggest eliminating things that sometimes trigger or aggravate canker sores, such as alcohol, chewing gum, citrus fruits, coffee, dairy products, meat, pineapple, spicy foods, tomatoes, toothpaste and vinegar and other acidic foods. (If you're not sure which foods are acidic, just put anything that tastes sour on the list.)

I'm all for using ice and rinsing your mouth with saltwater. And I think it's a great idea—as well as obvious—to avoid possible canker sore triggers whenever possible. I myself would also try these herbal alternatives.

★★ **Soothe your mouth with myrrh.** Myrrh is more than just a folk remedy for canker sores. Germany's Commission E, the body of scientists that provides advice on herbal matters, has endorsed powdered myrrh for the treatment of mild inflammations of the mouth and throat because it contains high amounts of tannins.

Tannin, the common name for tannic acid, is a constituent of many plants and gives foods an astringent taste. An antiseptic with broad-spectrum antibacterial and antiviral action, it's especially helpful for treating mouth sores, which could be caused by a bacterium, a fungus, a virus or an allergy.

To use powdered myrrh, just open a capsule (available at health food stores) and dab a little directly on the sore.

★★ **Try a tea bag.** Myrrh isn't the only herb that's high in tannin: Regular beverage tea also has a rich supply. Try placing a spent tea bag on your canker sores. Or make tea from some of the other herbs that are high in tannin, such as bearberry, eucalyptus, St.-John's-wort, sage, raspberry, peppermint and licorice.

★ **Consider cankerroot.** This plant got its name because of its traditional use as a treatment for canker sores. American Indians and early settlers alike used cankerroot as a tea to treat both sore throat and canker sores. Penobscot Indians chewed raw root for canker sores and fever blisters.

The plant, which is also known as goldthread, shares many of the active ingredients and healing properties of the more familiar goldenseal, barberry and Oregon grape.

Carpal Tunnel Syndrome

Carpal tunnel syndrome (CTS) is considered a repetitive motion injury—cumulative trauma associated with constant rapid use of the fingers (low-intensity, high-frequency finger work). CTS has been around for decades, the occupational hazard of bookkeepers and supermarket checkout clerks who punched buttons all day long. But it did not become a household word until the 1980s, when personal computers came to dominate so many workplaces. Suddenly, millions of people's jobs required the kind of steady, rapid finger movements that can cause repetitive motion injuries like CTS. It is also a problem for some musicians, factory workers and other people who must constantly use their hands.

Fortunately, there are quite a few herbs that can help alleviate this problem.

★★ **Drink lots of camomile tea.** Camomile tea is best known as a tasty way to calm jangled nerves. But its active compounds (bisabolol, chamazulene and cyclic ethers) also have potent anti-inflammatory action. Camomile is widely used in Europe for many inflammatory diseases. If I had CTS, I'd drink several cups of camomile tea a day.

★★ **Eat plenty of pineapple.** Pineapple contains a protein-dissolving (proteolytic) enzyme, bromelain, that is often recommended for CTS.

"Bromelain has well-documented effects on virtually all inflammatory conditions, regardless of cause," according to naturopaths Joseph Pizzorno, N.D., president of Bastyr University in Seattle, and Michael Murray, N.D., co-authors of *A Textbook of Natural Medicine.* "Bromelain can reduce swelling, inflammation and pain. Bromelain is extremely safe to use. In human studies, very large doses (nearly two grams) have been given without side effects."

Naturopaths suggest taking 250 to 1,500 milligrams of pure bromelain a day, between meals, to treat inflammatory conditions such as CTS. Bromelain is available at many health food stores. Since I favor food sources, however, I prefer to get my bromelain from pineapple itself. Ginger and papaya also contain helpful proteolytic enzymes. You might enjoy a Proteolytic CTS Fruit Salad composed of pineapple and papaya and spiced with grated ginger.

★★ **Season foods with turmeric.** This herb contains curcumin, a potent anti-inflammatory chemical. Some studies suggest that curcumin is only about half as effective as the pharmaceutical anti-inflammatory medication cortisone, but consider that cortisone is expensive and can have nasty side effects. Turmeric is much easier on the system and the pocketbook, not to mention a lot tastier.

Naturopaths suggest taking 250 to 500 milligrams of pure curcumin a day, between meals. Dried turmeric contains about 1 to 4 percent curcumin, so to get the dose that naturopaths recommend, you would have to consume 10 to 50 grams (5 to 25 teaspoons) of dried turmeric. That's a lot more than even I would add to a curried rice dish. Instead, try using turmeric liberally on food and then taking some more in capsules.

Colds and Flu

The common cold, an infection of the upper respiratory tract, is caused by any of 200 different viruses. The viral infection and the immune system's battle against it produce the all-too-familiar symptoms: sore throat, nasal congestion, runny nose, watery eyes, hacking cough and sometimes fever.

Colds are spread directly from person to person by coughing or sneezing or by hand-to-hand contact. The virus gets on one person's hands and can spread to the hands of others. If your virus-contaminated hands touch your nose or eyes, you catch the cold. The virus can also live for several hours on everyday surfaces like counters and doorknobs. Your hands can literally pick it up that way as well. (That's a good reason to wash your hands often during cold and flu season.)

The average American adult suffers two to three colds a year; the average young child has as many as nine. That adds up to something like one billion colds a year.

If you are getting more than your fair share of colds, your immune system may need help. Maybe the right herbs can help you as they have me. I definitely take these herbs, and I catch fewer colds than my wife and kids and grandkids.

There are quite a few herbs that can help boost your immune system's cold-fighting power.

★★★ **Reinforce your defenses with echinacea.** I use echinacea, also known as coneflower, myself. There's good research, most of it German, to show that it strengthens the immune system against cold viruses and many other germs as well. Echinacea increases levels of a chemical in the body called properdin, which activates the part of the immune system responsible for increasing defense mechanisms against viruses and bacteria.

Echinacea root extracts also possess antiviral activity against influenza, herpes and other viruses. In a study of 180 people with flu, one scientist found that 900 milligrams of an echinacea extract significantly reduced symptoms.

There's one odd thing about good echinacea: Shortly after ingesting a tea or tincture, it makes the tongue numb or tingly. Don't worry, though: This reaction is harmless.

But as effective as echinacea can be, it's no miracle cold cure. Even if you take this herb on a regular basis, you still might catch some colds. In fact, some herbalists caution that you should not use echinacea every day as an immune-enhancing tonic but should take it only when you feel a cold coming on or when those close to you have one. I'm still debating with myself on this.

★★★ **Battle bugs with garlic.** Eat enough garlic, and most people (along with their cold germs) will stay away from you. I'm just joking, and there really are some excellent reasons to use this herb to prevent colds and flu. Garlic contains several helpful compounds, including allicin, one of the plant kingdom's most potent, broad-spectrum antibiotics.

As anyone who has ever had garlic breath knows, this herb's aromatic compounds are readily released from the lungs and respiratory tract, putting garlic's active ingredients right where they can be most effective against cold viruses.

★★★ **Ease symptoms with ginger.** Pouring a cup of boiling water onto a couple of tablespoons of fresh, shredded ginger root to make a good hot tea really makes a lot of sense as a cold treatment. That's because this herb contains nearly a dozen antiviral compounds.

Scientists have isolated several chemicals (sesquiterpenes) in ginger that have specific effects against the most common family of cold viruses, the rhinoviruses. Some of these chemicals are remarkably potent in their anti-rhinovirus effects.

Still other constituents in ginger, gingerols and shogaols, help relieve cold symptoms because they reduce pain and fever, suppress coughing and have a mild sedative effect that encourages rest.

Ginger has one more thing going for it—it's tasty. I'd say there are a lot of good reasons to make ginger a regular part of your cold-treatment arsenal.

Constipation

Here's a sure-fire formula to create a problem with constipation: Take all the fiber-rich fruits, vegetables and whole grains out of your diet. In their place eat lots of meats, fats and dairy foods. No wonder an estimated 10 percent of Americans suffer from constipation, with at least 20 percent of the elderly complaining of it.

When I say that diet can control constipation, I'm not just talking about prune juice. Every whole-grain item and every fiber-rich fruit and vegetable helps prevent and relieve constipation. In folk medicine the foods that get special recognition as laxatives include almonds, apples, avocados, chicory, dandelion, dates, endive, figs, flaxseed, grapes, mangos, papayas, parsley, persimmons, pineapple, prunes, rhubarb, rutabagas, soybeans, turnips, walnuts and watercress. You might easily contrive any number of soups and salads from this list.

If you are constipated, the first thing you should do is change your diet to the "double high five" by eating five fruits and five vegetables a day. If you are still constipated after two days, increase your fruit and veggie intake while diminishing your intake of low-fiber foods like meats and refined breads. Also, I'd recommend that you avoid tea if constipation is a problem for you. Tea is rich in tannins, which is one reason that it is recommended as a treatment for diarrhea. Tannins help bind stools and hold back bowel movements.

Fruit and vegetable juices also work, especially those that retain much of their fiber. Prune juice tops the list, of course, but some juice advocates say that apple-pear juice is a particularly good laxative. Among vegetable juices, asparagus, jícama and potato have been suggested.

Some people who favor juicing use machines that eject most of the fiber. When it comes to treating constipation, that's a big mistake, because fiber is precisely what you want.

Several herbs can also help prevent and treat constipation.

★★ **Favor flaxseed.** Also known as linseed, flaxseed as an herbal treatment for constipation gets an endorsement from Commission E, the body of scientists that provides advice on herbal treatments to Germany's equivalent of the Food and Drug Administration. Commission E suggests taking one to three tablespoons of whole or crushed flaxseed two or three times a day for chronic constipation.

A special word of warning: If you try this remedy, make sure that you also get plenty of water—at least eight full glasses a day—to keep all that bulk moving through your digestive system.

★★ **Take psyllium for extra fiber.** Tiny psyllium seeds contain a fiber called mucilage, which absorbs a great deal of fluid in the gut. This makes the seeds swell. They add bulk to stool, and as stool becomes bulkier, it presses on the colon wall, triggering the muscle contractions we experience as "the urge." Psyllium is quite popular in Germany, and Commission E approves taking three to ten tablespoons a day for chronic constipation.

As with flaxseed, psyllium needs water to work, and if you take it without water, it might obstruct your digestive tract.

And if you have asthma, don't take this herb. There have been several reports of allergic reactions to psyllium, including a few serious asthma attacks from inhaled seed dust.

You should also watch how you react to this herb if you have allergies. If allergic symptoms develop after you take it once, don't use it again.

★ **Turn to rhubarb.** I like this constipation-relief recipe from physician Ronald Hoffman, M.D., that was published in *Parade* magazine: Puree three stalks of rhubarb without the leaves. Add one cup of apple juice, a quarter of a peeled lemon and one tablespoon of honey. It will make a thick, tart drink that should do the trick.

Dr. Hoffman is right about rhubarb. It contains a natural laxative chemical. It's also high in fiber. Remember, though, that its laxative action can be pretty powerful; you should probably try some other methods first.

Corns

Corns are hardened, mound-shaped areas of increased growth on the skin of the toes. Hard corns occur on the toes, while soft corns arise between the toes.

The best way to deal with corns is to prevent them from forming in the first place. Almost always, they're caused by shoes that fit too tightly, bunching up the toes and irritating the skin. Many people, especially women, wear shoes that are too small for them in the belief that small feet make them appear daintier. But in my opinion, the pain just isn't worth it. (Personally, I'd rather be with a happy, healthy woman in shoes that fit her than with a woman who cripples herself in the name of daintiness.)

If you can't prevent corns, then I'd suggest some herbal treatments that should help.

★ **Treat your feet with fruit.** When King Solomon developed boils, his physicians applied figs; this is one of the very few descriptions of the medicinal use of herbs in the Bible. Figs contain protein-dissolving enzymes that help dissolve unwanted skin growths, including corns. Papaya and pineapple contain similar enzymes, and all three fruits have age-old reputations for reducing corns and warts.

Here's a recipe culled from my database that I might try if I ever abandoned my barefoot ways and got a corn. Open a fresh fig and tape the pulp to the corn overnight. Or cut a square of pineapple peel and tape the inner side to the corn overnight. The following morning, remove the tape and soak the foot in hot water. After an hour or so, try to remove the corn. It should come off fairly easily, but you can rub it gently with a pumice stone if necessary.

"Some stubborn cases, however, may require four to five overnight treatments," warns medical anthropologist John Heinerman, Ph.D., author of *Heinerman's Encyclopedia of Fruits, Vegetables and Herbs*. Folklore attests to some fairly similar procedures using papaya.

★ **Dissolve corns with willow.** Willow contains aspirin-like compounds known as salicylates that relieve pain. But salicylates are also powerful acids that can help dissolve corns and warts. Just use this herb carefully, placing willow bark poultices directly on the corn itself; don't let the herb come in contact with the surrounding skin. Because they're acidic, salicylates may cause skin inflammation.

★ **Warm up to wintergreen.** This is another good source of salicylates. Some herbalists recommend that you apply wintergreen oil to remove calluses, corns, cysts and warts. I'd probably try it for corns, both to dissolve hardened skin and to relieve pain. Again, to make sure you avoid irritation, apply the oil only to the corn itself and not to the surrounding skin.

Remember, though, to keep wintergreen oil (or any product containing it) out of the reach of children. The minty smell can be very tempting, but ingesting even small amounts can prove fatal to young children.

Coughing

The common cough is perhaps more common than the common cold. Roughly half of the people seeking medical care in winter suffer from inflammation of the respiratory tract, with cough and other related symptoms. No matter what the cause, coughing is pretty much the same—productive coughs bring up mucus, while nonproductive or dry, hacking coughs do not.

Remember, if you have a cough that just won't go away, it means that your body is sending you some kind of message. It could be something as simple as "stop smoking" or "get that sinus infection cleared up." While you're treating your cough, you also need to pay attention to what your body is trying to tell you. If home remedies don't seem to help and your cough persists for several days, see your doctor.

Regardless of the cause, however, herbs can provide some relief. Herbal cough treatments have been recommended since ancient times. Here are some that I'd recommend.

★★ **Evade problems with elderberry.** Israeli scientists praise elderberry for treating colds, cough and fever. An Israeli study showed that a drug (Sambucol, which is now available in the United States) made from elderberry is effective against flu, including the cough that goes with it. You can also purchase an elderberry tincture or use the dried herb to make a tea. I would not hesitate to use American elderberry instead.

★★ **Quiet your cough with ginger.** Several chemicals in ginger (gingerols and shogaols) have been shown in studies using laboratory animals to have cough-suppressing, pain-relieving and fever-reducing action. Similar effects in humans have not been demonstrated, but I believe that ginger can help relieve a cough. You can try adding it to whatever you take for coughs.

★★ **Clear your throat with lemonade.** Here's a cough formula from Christopher Hobbs, a fourth-generation California herbalist and author of several fine books on herbal medicines: Steep 2 teaspoons of organic lemon rinds, 1 teaspoon of sage and ½ teaspoon of thyme in boiling water for 15 minutes. Then add the juice of ½ lemon and 1 tablespoon of honey. I'm quite partial to lemonade, and I think this remedy is definitely worth trying. In fact, drink it two or three times a day. (Hobbs calls for organic rinds because it is just about impossible to wash away the pesticides that are commonly used on citrus fruits.)

Cuts, Scrapes, and Abscesses

Everyone develops skin infections of one kind or another at some point in life. If a cut becomes more red, tender or painful after a day or two or starts oozing fluid, it means that you have an infection that should be treated by a doctor.

Here are several herbs that can be very effective in treating minor cuts. If you'd like to try them on more serious cuts and abscesses (they do work), please discuss it with your physician before doing so.

★★★ **Apply a natural antiseptic.** Teatree oil was used by Australian aborigines and early settlers to treat abrasions, athlete's foot, bug bites, burns and cuts. Its use as a wound treatment has spread around the world. There's good reason for this, as it contains the powerful antiseptic compound terpinen-4-ol.

Varro Tyler, Ph.D., dean and professor emeritus of pharmacognosy (natural product pharmacy) at Purdue University in West Lafayette, Indiana, recommends teatree oil as a wound treatment.

I have personally used teatree oil as an externally applied antiseptic for abscesses, and I can attest to its value. It is well-proven as an antiseptic against bacteria and fungi. In fact, teatree oil is just as good as any of those nonherbal antiseptics Mother used to use—iodine and mercurochrome.

People who are sensitive to it may find that the pure oil irritates their skin. I suggest diluting it by putting several drops in a couple of tablespoons of any vegetable oil. If you find that the oil irritates your skin, dilute it further or discontinue use. And don't take teatree oil, or any essential oils, internally. They are extremely concentrated, and even small quantities of many of them can be poisonous.

★★ **Make a calendula compress.** Commission E, the expert committee of German medicinal herb experts that advises the German government, endorses calendula for reducing inflammation and promoting wound healing. It does both.

To make a wash to treat cuts, pour a cup of boiling water over a teaspoon of dry petals and steep for ten minutes. Then soak a clean cloth in the liquid and apply it as a compress on the wound.

Calendula may be even more effective in creams. You can buy commercial skin treatment products containing calendula in many health food stores.

★★ **Stimulate healing with comfrey.** This herb contains a compound, allantoin, that helps heal wounds. Its astringent tannic acids may also contribute to wound healing.

Comfrey has gotten some bad press recently because it contains chemicals called pyrrolizidine alkaloids, which can damage the liver. Many authorities warn against ingesting it. But there's little if any risk in applying comfrey externally. It's still my first line of defense against sores that are slow to heal. To use it, you can take some fresh leaves and rub them directly on the affected area. You can also find commercial skin-care products containing comfrey in many health food stores.

Dandruff

Dandruff is a common scalp condition that causes unsightly white flakes to appear in the scalp and hair. The white flakes are dead scalp skin. Dandruff is often the result of seborrhea, an inflammation (dermatitis) of the scalp. Here are some herbs you might try for preventing and treating dandruff.

★★★ **Fill up on biotin-rich foods.** Biotin is an important vitamin-like nutrient that the body uses in many ways. While there seems to be some biotin in just about all plants, my database reveals some standouts. Soybeans have the most, followed by garlic, American ginseng, oats, barley, Asian ginseng, avocado, cottonseed, alfalfa, sesame, corn, fava beans and elderberry.

Lamentably, my database can't provide the whole story, because science just doesn't know all that much about the biotin content of plants. That's due to the amazing fact that no one has ever been funded to do detailed analyses of the minor constituents of all those fruits, nuts and veggies that the government is urging us to consume. (You might want to contact your Congressional representative to request funding for more detailed nutritional studies.)

★ **Control flaking with comfrey.** Allantoin, a chemical in this herb, has anti-dandruff properties, according to *Hunting's Encyclopedia of Shampoo Ingredients*. You might be able to find a commercial shampoo that contains comfrey at a health food store. If not, you can add a couple of drops of comfrey tincture to your favorite herbal shampoo.

★ **Try the Egyptian cure.** Medical anthropologist John Heinerman, Ph.D., author of *Heinerman's Encyclopedia of Fruits, Vegetables and Herbs*, shares the following Egyptian dandruff/seborrhea treatment: Take one to two tablespoons of ginger juice (squeezed from about two grated roots) and mix it with three tablespoons of sesame oil and a half-teaspoon of lemon juice. Rub the mixture into the scalp three times a week. I think it sounds interesting, although sesame oil can be expensive. If I had dandruff, I might give this one a try.

Depression

It goes without saying that everyone gets the blues from time to time. Depression that won't let up, however, is a serious disorder. If you suffer from ongoing depression, you should see your doctor for treatment. In the meantime, there are also a number of herbs that can prove helpful.

★★★ **Let licorice boost your mood.** No plant in my database has more anti-depressant compounds than licorice, but it does not have St.-John's-wort's folk history of use as an antidepressant. Strange. At least eight licorice compounds are monoamine oxidase (MAO) inhibitors, which are compounds capable of potent antidepressant action.

If you'd like to try licorice to beat depression, simply add some to any of the other herbal teas suggested in this chapter. (While licorice and its extracts are safe for normal use in moderate amounts—up to about three cups of tea a day—long-term use or ingestion of larger amounts can produce headache, lethargy, sodium and water retention, excessive loss of potassium and high blood pressure.)

★★★ **Sample St.-John's-wort.** This herb got its name because the plant flowers on St. John's day, June 24. (*Wort* is Old English for "plant.") Its star-shaped yellow flowers, which turn red when bruised, are beautiful enough to make anyone with the blues feel happier. But this herb also has a long history of folk use for treating anxiety and depression. Modern science has shown that generations of folk herbalists were right.

Clinical studies show that treatment with just one of the active compounds in this herb, hypericin, results in significant improvement in anxiety, depression and feelings of worthlessness. Some studies show that it's a more powerful anti-depressant than some pharmaceutical drugs such as amitriptyline (Elavil) and imiprimine (Tofranil). What's more, it has fewer side effects. Some researchers say that it has no side effects at all.

Studies also show that St.-John's-wort improves sleep quality, often a major problem for people who are seriously depressed. In one study, German researchers gave St.-John's-wort to 105 people with moderate depression. Compared with a similar group not receiving the herb, they slept better and exhibited less sadness, helplessness, hopelessness, exhaustion and headache. They also reported no side effects.

★★ **Banish the blues with purslane.** Many people get the urge to eat when they are depressed. And eating just might help—if you eat the right foods. Foods containing the minerals magnesium and potassium have been shown to have antidepressant effects. Purslane, which is very rich in these minerals, is also high in other constituents with antidepressant value, including calcium, folate (the naturally occurring form of folic acid) and lithium. In fact, purslane contains up to a whopping 16 percent antidepressant compounds, figured on a dry-weight basis.

Working with my database, it's clear that purslane is just one of several salad ingredients that might help relieve depression. Hence, my Un-Sad Salad: lettuce, pigweed, purslane, lamb's-quarters and watercress. I'd also be sure to use a little thyme in the dressing, as it's very high in the antidepressant mineral lithium.

Diarrhea

Everyone knows what diarrhea is. Many serious diseases can cause it. And infectious diarrhea, caused by viruses or bacteria, still ranks as a leading killer of Third World children. But this chapter is devoted to common, run-of-the-mill diarrhea that usually clears up within 48 hours.

The most important thing to do for diarrhea is to drink fluids, but a lot of people do just the opposite. They cut down in the mistaken belief that refraining from drinking fluids will help the body stop producing them. The fact is, the main medical risk of ordinary diarrhea is dehydration. So keep getting fluids by sipping water or astringent iced tea throughout the day.

There are a number of herbal approaches to clearing up a bout of diarrhea. All of these herbs contain one or more of three natural ingredients: tannin, pectin and mucilage.

Tannins are the chemicals that give some herbs their astringency—that is, the ability to bind up or contract tissues. Tannins' astringent action reduces intestinal inflammation. The tannins bind to the protein layer of the inflamed mucous membranes and cause them to thicken, hence slowing resorption of toxic materials and restricting secretions.

Pectin is a soluble fiber that adds bulk to stool and soothes the gut. The "pectate" in the over-the-counter antidiarrheal medicine Kaopectate contains pectin.

Mucilage soothes the digestive tract and adds bulk to stool by absorbing water and swelling considerably.

Here are several of the many herbs that can be helpful.

★ **Sip a cup of agrimony tea.** Commission E endorses agrimony for common diarrhea, probably due to its high tannin content. Try using two to three teaspoons of leaves to make a tea.

★ **Eat some applesauce.** Apple pulp is rich in pectin. That's why apples and applesauce are a hallowed folk remedy for diarrhea. (Apple pectin also helps treat constipation because it acts as a gentle stool softener. Like psyllium, it's amphoteric, which means that it works in either direction, plugging you up if your bowels are loose or loosening you up if you are constipated.)

★ **Soothe your bowels with berries.** Commission E, the body of scientists that advises the German government about herbs, suggests making an astringent tea with two teaspoons of blackberry leaf. Oddly, it does not mention raspberry leaf, which is a close botanical relative that is also high in tannin. I've used both and found them effective.

Diverticulitis

Our ancestors ate lots of fiber, and our colons evolved to handle it. Without enough fiber, we know, strange things begin to happen down there. Food moves more slowly through the colon, causing constipation, and little pockets known as diverticula develop in the colon wall. Sometimes diverticula become plugged with little bits of digested food and often little seeds. If diverticula become inflamed and swell, they cause pain and the other symptoms of diverticulitis.

More than half of those over 60 have noninflamed, painless diverticula, while an estimated 10 percent develop the inflammation of diverticulitis.

To reduce your risk of diverticulitis, the two most important factors are a high-fiber diet and exercise, according to Walid H. Aldoori, M.D., professor in the Department of Nutrition at the Harvard School of Public Health. But while you're eating more whole grains and fresh fruits and vegetables, you should watch some other dietary factors as well. Be sure to drink plenty of nonalcoholic fluids to keep things moving efficiently through your digestive tract. And if you've had diverticulitis, you should steer clear of some small, indigestible seeds—poppy, sesame, raspberry and strawberry—which can plug diverticula and aggravate the condition.

There are many herbs that can help. Here are my favorites.

★★★ **Learn to be flax-ible.** Commission E, the German expert panel that passes on the safety, effectiveness and dosage of medicinal herbs for the German government, approves using one to three tablespoons of crushed flaxseed two or three times a day (with lots of water) to treat diverticulitis.

★★★ **Get extra fiber from psyllium.** Powdery, high-fiber psyllium seed is the major ingredient in Metamucil and a few other bulk-forming commercial laxatives. A few tablespoons a day (with plenty of water) provide a healthy amount of diverticulitis-preventing fiber. Watch how you react to this herb if you have allergies, however. If allergic symptoms develop after you take it once, don't use it again.

★★ **Give discomfort the slip.** Andrew Weil, M.D., professor at the University of Arizona College of Medicine in Tucson and author of *Natural Health, Natural Medicine*, suggests using slippery elm bark powder to treat diverticulitis. The fibrous bark contains large quantities of a gentle laxative that soothes the digestive tract while keeping things moving.

The Food and Drug Administration has declared slippery elm to be a safe and effective digestive soother. Prepare it like oatmeal, adding hot milk or water to the powdered bark to make a cereal.

Dizziness

The terms *dizziness* and *vertigo* are often used interchangeably, but technically there is a distinction. Dizziness simply means unsteadiness. Vertigo is worse. It is a disorienting illusion of movement, as if the world were whirling around you, or you around it.

If you have chronic dizziness, see a physician. Prolonged or recurring bouts of dizziness can be a sign of inner ear infection, cardiac arryhthmia, high blood pressure or some other serious problems. For occasional bouts of dizziness, there are several herbs that might prove helpful.

★★★ **Make a motion in favor of ginger.** Chinese sailors chewed ginger root for seasickness thousands of years ago, and as they traveled, their remedy did, too—from Asia to India to the Middle East and on to Europe.

"To prevent motion sickness, swallow two capsules 30 minutes before departure and then one to two more as symptoms begin to occur, probably about every four hours," suggests Varro Tyler, Ph.D., dean and professor emeritus of pharmacognosy (natural product pharmacy) at Purdue University in West Lafayette, Indiana. Ginger capsules are available at health food stores and other supplement outlets.

You can also try fresh ginger tea or slices of candied ginger, according to herb advocate Andrew Weil, M.D., professor at the University of Arizona College of Medicine in Tucson and author of *Natural Health, Natural Medicine*.

★★ **Give ginkgo a whirl.** Ginkgo extract is prescribed extensively in Europe for vertigo, among many other conditions. One French study of 70 people with chronic vertigo showed that 47 percent improved while taking ginkgo. You can try 60 to 240 milligrams a day, but don't go any higher than that. In large amounts, ginkgo may cause diarrhea, irritability and restlessness.

★ **Capitalize on celery.** Celery seed has a long history of use in traditional Chinese medicine as a treatment for dizziness.

Dry Mouth

Dry mouth is not only uncomfortable, it's also not good for you. Saliva helps control bacteria populations in the mouth, and in doing so it helps prevent tooth decay, gum disease and mouth infections.

An estimated 25 percent of older Americans complain of dry mouth. The condition is common among public speakers like me, hence the inevitable water glass at the podium. It is also related to aging and is a side effect of more than 400 widely used medications, including many prescribed for high blood pressure and depression.

In addition, dry mouth is a symptom of Sjögren's syndrome, a condition often associated with rheumatoid arthritis that also causes dry eyes.

If you're ever caught with dry mouth, sip water frequently, especially when eating or speaking. Avoid coffee and sugary beverages, both of which can aggravate dry mouth. Also avoid alcohol, tobacco and salty foods. In addition, try these herbs.

★ **Stimulate saliva with echinacea.** One compound in echinacea, echinacein, is a proven saliva producer. I recommend taking a dropperful of tincture in juice. If you have access to the fresh plant, you can also chew the root. In addition to stimulating salivation, echinacea tends to numb the mouth, but this effect is temporary and harmless.

★ **Ease dryness with evening primrose.** Oil from the evening primrose is a rich source of a compound known as gamma-linolenic acid (GLA). Few reviewing the medical literature can have any doubts that GLA is a potent treatment for autoimmune disorders, which are caused by a confused immune system attacking the body itself. Sjögren's syndrome is thought to be an autoimmune disorder.

If I had dry mouth caused by Sjögren's, I would try evening primrose oil. You can buy capsules of the oil in natural food stores. Simply follow the package directions.

★ **Let rose come to your rescue.** In China, people simmer two to four teaspoons of dried multiflora rose flowers per cup of boiling water to make a tea for treating dry mouth.

Earache

Earache has many possible causes. In children, the most common by far is an infection that invades the middle ear—what doctors call otitis media. But earache can also be caused by excess earwax, a perforated eardrum and other conditions in the head and neck. There's also an outer ear infection called otitis externa.

Earache treatment begins with pain relief and then proceeds to dealing with the cause. Physicians treat the pain with acetaminophen (or aspirin for adults), then give antibiotics and decongestants to treat the infection itself.

Do not give either aspirin or its natural herbal alternatives to children who develop ear infections along with colds. When children take aspirin-like drugs for viral infections (especially colds, flu and chicken pox), there's a chance that they might get Reye's syndrome, a potentially fatal condition that damages the liver and brain. This herbalist hates to say it, but if my grandkids developed ear infections from colds, I'd treat their ear pain with acetaminophen rather than herbal relatives of aspirin.

Once you've treated the pain, it's time to consider the cause. A doctor can look in the affected ear and decide if you have an external or an internal problem.

There are a number of herbs that can help alleviate the pain of earache or treat the causes.

★ **Pamper your ear with echinacea.** Echinacea, also known as coneflower, has both antibiotic and immune-boosting effects. You can try using a teaspoon of dried herb in tea or a dropperful of echinacea tincture in juice or tea. Drink either three times a day. I use echinacea to treat all sorts of infections, and I would probably try it if I had an earache. (Although echinacea can cause your tongue to tingle or go numb temporarily, this effect is harmless.)

★ **Take garlic to battle infection-causing bugs.** Like echinacea, garlic and its extracts have antibiotic and immune-boosting benefits. In studies, dripping garlic oil directly into the ear canal has been shown to treat fungal infections as well as or better than pharmaceutical drugs.

Taken internally, garlic can help cure a middle ear infection. If you have an earache, I suggest adding more garlic to your cooking. You might also try putting a few drops of garlic oil in the painful ear.

★ **Try an herbal trio.** Some naturopaths suggest using a mixture of echinacea, goldenseal and licorice root (this just for flavor). You can make a tea using either a teaspoon of each herb or a dropperful of each tincture per cup of boiling water. Enjoy a cup three times a day.

Although I don't have proof that this mixture is superior to either echinacea or goldenseal alone, I suspect that the combination of herbs is a better treatment.

Erection Problems

Not long ago, doctors and psychologists believed that 90 percent of erection difficulties were psychological and that a stimulating partner was all a man needed. Now authorities agree that most erection impairment has a physical cause: clogged arteries, alcohol or other drugs, diabetes, pelvic injuries, sleep deprivation, smoking or prostate surgery.

Impotence is the inability to raise or sustain an erection that is adequate for intercourse and ejaculation. Some 30 million American men experience some form of impotence, with more than a million currently being treated. Some take prescription medication, such as Viagra. Others get penile implants. The newest approach involves self-injecting a hormone known as prostaglandin E. Within a few minutes, it produces a 90-minute erection.

But before you go sticking needles into your penis, you might try some of these herbal approaches.

★★★ **Favor the fava bean.** Alleged to have incited the ancient Roman poet Cicero to passion, the fava bean is our best food source of the compound L-dopa, which is often used to treat Parkinson's disease. Large amounts of L-dopa may cause priapism, a painful, persistent erection that has nothing to do with sexual arousal.

I wouldn't advocate doses of L-dopa large enough to cause priapism, but you'd be hard put to eat enough fava beans to ever cause a problem. Fava beans have an age-old reputation as an aphrodisiac. I suspect that a big serving—8 to 16 ounces—just might contain enough L-dopa to give erection a nice boost.

If fava beans seem to help, try sprouting them. The sprouts contain even more L-dopa.

★★★ **Boost blood flow with ginkgo.** Ginkgo is best known for improving blood flow through the brain. But it also seems to boost blood flow into the penis, thus aiding iffy erections.

In several small studies, physicians have obtained very good results with 60 to 240 milligrams daily of a standardized ginkgo extract. In one nine-month study, 78 percent of men with impotence due to atherosclerotic clogging of the penile artery reported significant improvement without side effects.

People normally think of atherosclerosis as a disease that clogs the blood vessels that supply the heart, thereby leading to heart attacks. This same disease can also clog the blood vessels that supply the penis and lead to erection problems.

In another six-month study, half of the men being treated with ginkgo regained their erections. The active compounds are too dilute in ginkgo leaves to do much good, so standardized extracts concentrate it: A 50:1 extract means that 50 pounds of leaves were used to produce 1 pound of extract. These extracts are available at many health food stores and herb shops.

You can try 60 to 240 milligrams a day, but don't go any higher than that. In large amounts, ginkgo may cause diarrhea, irritability and restlessness. And do give it time to work. In about six months, you'll know whether it's going to do the trick.

★★★ **Discover the velvet bean.** Years ago, while working in Panama, I was told by more than one informant that the seeds of the velvet or ox-eye bean (in Spanish, *ojo de buey*) were aphrodisiac. That was before I knew that these seeds can contain as much L-dopa as fava beans, and perhaps more.

Fever

While people rightly regard fever as a sign of infection, attempting to bring it down is sometimes a mistake. Up to a point, fever is a friend. Most microorganisms that cause disease die when exposed to high temperatures, so fever is one of the ways in which the immune system tries to kill them. The trouble is that prolonged high fevers can kill us, too.

A good rule of thumb is: Don't treat every fever right away. Treat it when it starts making you feel uncomfortable. For high fever—above 103°F—you'll want to consult a doctor as soon as possible, of course. For milder high temperature—99° to 101°F—you may choose to take aspirin, acetaminophen or ibuprofen (Motrin or Advil). One word of caution: Most benign fevers start to let up within a day or two. If any fever, even a mild one, persists for more than 48 hours, see your doctor.

There are a number of herbs that can help reduce a fever. As a general rule, however, remember that it's not a good idea to give aspirin or aspirin-like herbs to children who have fevers with viral infections such as colds, flu and chicken pox. There is a chance that they could develop Reye's syndrome, a potentially fatal condition that causes liver and brain damage. And if you are allergic to aspirin, you probably shouldn't use aspirin-like herbs.

★★★ **To lower your temperature, sip willow bark tea.** When the eighteenth-century British minister Edward Stone set out to find a cheap substitute for expensive imported cinchona bark, which was used to treat malaria and other fevers, he noticed that willow bark tasted just as bitter and decided to try it.

Willow proved to be a good pain reliever and fever fighter, and its use spread around England, Europe and the Americas. The active compound salicin was isolated in 1830, and the Bayer company tinkered with salicin to create aspirin. The new Bayer Aspirin was released in the 1890s, and it quickly became one of the world's most popular drugs. But you can still use willow bark. I do.

Try making a tea with one to two teaspoons of dried bark steeped in a cup of boiling water for about 20 minutes. You can mask the bitter taste with cinnamon, ginger, camomile or other flavorful herbs.

★★ **Beat the heat with meadowsweet.** This is another excellent source of salicin, the chemical in willow bark that fights fever. Commission E, the body of experts that advises the German government about herbs, suggests making a tea with one to two teaspoons of meadowsweet flowers. Try up to three cups a day.

Flatulence

Most gas, or flatus, is produced in the intestine by undigested carbohydrates. Instead of being broken down in the stomach, some starches enter the small intestine intact. The intestine does not produce the enzymes necessary to digest two specific carbohydrates, raffinose and stachyose, so they just sit there until the bacteria that normally inhabit the bowel ferment them, a process that releases gas.

Guess which foods are highest in raffinose and stachyose? You guessed it—beans. And among beans, the three that are highest in that pair of carbohydrates are English peas, soybeans and black-eyed peas. But those aren't the only ones: Limas, pintos, black beans and other legumes also contain enough of these indigestible carbohydrates to produce gas.

If you think that you're producing more gas than you used to, you may be right. If you've evolved your diet in a healthier direction recently and are eating less meat, fewer fats and more carbohydrates (especially beans), the chances are that you've been eating more of the foods that are most likely to produce gas.

Most people who complain of "excess gas," on the other hand, actually produce amounts that digestive system specialists (gastroenterologists) would call perfectly normal. Studies show that the average adult passes gas from 8 to 20 times every waking hour of the day. In other words, there's nothing unusual about releasing gas more than once an hour.

Just because flatulence is normal doesn't mean it's welcome. Flatus cannot be banished from the body, but you can significantly reduce the likelihood of unwanted exclamations. A number of herbs can help.

★★★ **Curb emissions with carminatives.** Any herb that soothes the digestive tract and has a reputation for minimizing flatus is known as a carminative. Dozens of herbs fall into this category, so it's hard to highlight just a few. The most helpful are those containing the most gas-relieving chemicals, most notably the compounds camphor, carvone, eugenol, menthol and thymol. These compounds are especially concentrated in allspice, cloves, cornmint, caraway, dill, fennel, horsebalm, peppermint, sage and thyme.

In addition, most of the herbs in the mint and carrot families are good carminatives, including aniseed, basil, bergamot, camomile, cinnamon, coriander, garlic, ginger, hyssop, juniper, lavender, lemon, marjoram, nutmeg, onion, oregano, rosemary, savory and tarragon. Try using carminative herbs to flavor starchy dishes, especially those made with beans.

You can also deflate flatus with my Carminatea, made with camomile, caraway, dill, fennel, lemon balm (also known as melissa) and peppermint and sweetened with licorice.

Gingivitis

Gingivitis means "inflammation of the gums." It causes swelling, redness, a change in normal gum contours, watery discharge and bleeding. When it gets more serious, it becomes pyorrhea, degeneration of the gum tissue supporting the teeth. Together, gingivitis and pyorrhea are known as periodontal disease, a problem that all of us are more likely to have as we get older.

At age 10, about 15 percent of Americans have at least a mild form of gingivitis. At age 20, some 38 percent have it, and at 50, about half. People who don't brush, floss or get regular dental care are at greatest risk.

But you can get gingivitis even if you do brush and floss, because brushing and flossing don't clean out the deep, bacteria-harboring pockets between the teeth and gums. For those areas you need a little extra help.

Dentists treat gingivitis by irrigating the deep pockets with antiseptics. But if you want an alternative route to gum care, here are some herbs that can also help.

★★ **Kill bacteria with bloodroot.** My advocacy of the compound sanguinarine, found in bloodroot, is backed up by many well-designed studies. Research shows that toothpaste containing sanguinarine is modestly effective against several types of oral bacteria and that it helps reduce the amount of dental plaque in the mouth in as little as eight days.

If you'd like to try this herb, look for sanguinarine in the list of ingredients on the labels of toothpastes and mouthwashes. The most widely available brand is Viadent.

In addition to their use in over-the-counter products, bloodroot extracts are used by dentists to treat periodontal disease.

★★ **Gargle with camomile.** Commission E, the panel of experts that judges the safety and effectiveness of herbal medicines for the German government, considers camomile effective as a gargle or mouthwash for treating gingivitis. Camomile contains several anti-inflammatory and antiseptic compounds.

In addition to treating gum disease, you can use camomile to help prevent it. Try brewing a strong camomile tea using two to three teaspoons of herb per cup of boiling water. Steep for ten minutes, strain, and drink after meals. Or use it as a mouthwash. While ethnodentists caution that camomile, because it's kin to ragweed, may cause allergies, in my experience it is very rare. If you do notice an allergic reaction—itching or any discomfort—discontinue use of this herb.

★★ **Keep gums healthy with sage.** In the European herbal folk tradition, sage leaves, which are rather gritty, are rubbed on the gums and teeth as a stimulant dentifrice. I've done this, and it seems to help, thanks to sage's astringent tannin and several aromatic antiseptic compounds. I find sage leaves in my herb garden almost year-round, and collecting these leaves is a lot cheaper than buying products containing sanguinarine. Sage tea is perhaps as effective as a sanguinarine toothpaste.

Some modern research appears to support this folk medicine approach. Commission E endorses using two to three teaspoons of dried sage leaves per cup of boiling water to make an anti-gingivitis tea. It's best, though, to use sage in moderation, as it contains a fair amount of thujone, a compound that in very high doses may cause convulsions.

Gout

Gout is a form of arthritis because it causes pain in the joints, usually the big toe, although other joints can be affected. It's caused by a buildup of uric acid in the blood. When levels rise beyond a certain point, uric acid crystals form and collect in the affected joint or joints, causing excruciating pain. These crystals can also form in the body's major organs and do considerable damage, so avoiding pain is not the only reason to keep this serious condition under control.

Gout tends to run in families. Three hundred years ago, it was associated with wealth, because gout attacks were thought to be provoked by eating a rich diet. Now we know that the disease afflicts rich and poor alike. More than 95 percent of people who have gout are men over 30. An estimated 10 to 20 percent of the population has elevated uric acid levels, but only 3 people in 1,000 experience gout.

If you have gout, by all means take the medication that your doctor prescribes. But in addition, you might want to try some natural approaches to relieving this painful ailment.

★★★ **To reduce uric acid, count on celery seed.** Learning that celery extracts might help eliminate uric acid, I began taking two to four tablets of celery seed extracts daily instead of allopurinol. As I write, six months have gone by without a single gout crisis. For one week, I ate four celery stalks a day in lieu of the extracts.

These self-dosing anecdotal results lead me to believe the advertisement that led me to the celery seed. A skeptic then, I'm a believer now: Celery seed (or serendipity) has kept my uric acid below critical levels.

★★ **Get to know chiso.** This aromatic, weedy mint, imported accidentally or intentionally from Asia decades ago, is a popular food and medicine in the Orient. Here it's a rampant weed, but you'll find it grown intentionally behind some Japanese restaurants in the eastern United States.

Japanese researchers have touted compounds in chiso to relieve gout. It contains fairly high levels of four compounds known as xanthine oxidase (XO) inhibitors, which help prevent the synthesis of uric acid. I frequently add a little chiso to my mint teas, just as the Japanese add it to their sushi.

★★ **Pair chiso with licorice.** Like chiso, licorice contains several XO inhibitors, but at fairly low levels. Still, a chiso-licorice combo could be interesting, and the two herbs might even work better together.

Hangover

Hangover is a mild version of alcohol withdrawal syndrome. The headache is prompted in part by alcohol's relaxing effect on the blood vessels. As they open up, more blood flows through them, which causes the sensation of warmth we feel when drinking. But if the blood vessels of the head open too much, they trigger the pain nerves.

Alcohol is also a diuretic, so fluid loss contributes to morning-after thirst and can add to head pain.

The nausea and vomiting are a combination of alcohol's irritating effect on the stomach and its many effects on the central nervous system.

The fatigue and general lousy-all-over feeling result from alcohol's depressant effect and a buildup of acids in the blood (acidosis). The chemical acetaldehyde may also accumulate in the blood, leading to flushing.

Finally, additives and impurities in alcohol (congeners) contribute to hangovers. The general rule is that the darker the alcohol, the worse the hangover. Vodka and white wine contain few congeners, but bourbon, scotch and red wine are loaded with them.

I hate to state the obvious, but it needs to be said that a good basic approach to hangover is to prevent it by not drinking in the first place. Or you might try drinking clear liquor or white wine rather than the dark stuff. It also helps to drink lots of nonalcoholic beverages to stay well-hydrated and wash the acids out of your blood. All this helps head off both the headache and the upset stomach.

In addition, try these natural hangover aids.

★ **Brew some bitters.** The bitter bark that gives tonic water its flavor and is the source of quinine is used as a hangover remedy in China. Water in and of itself helps, but I suspect that bitter herbs like cinchona provide added benefit. Other bitter herbs often recommended for hangover include dandelion, gentian, mugwort and angostura, which is the same herb used in Angostura Bitters, a favorite hangover remedy among bartenders.

You can make an anti-hangover tea by adding a few drops of Angostura Bitters to a cup of boiling water. In fact, any of these herbs can be made into a very bitter tea. I'd suggest cutting the bitter flavor by adding the tasty herbs roselle and tamarind, both of which are also reputed to help banish hangover.

★ **Speed symptoms' departure with ginkgo.** Ginkgo seeds are not approved as food by the Food and Drug Administration, but they are available here. The Japanese have long served ginkgo seeds at cocktail parties, based on folklore assertions that they prevent drunkenness and hangover. Scientific studies out of Japan have shown that there is good reason to suspect that ginkgo seeds really can get the job done. It turns out that the seeds contain an enzyme that speeds up the body's metabolism of alcohol.

★ **To stop overimbibing, count on kudzu.** Some scientists finger a specific chemical (acetaldehyde) as the big culprit in hangover. Kudzu can cause acetaldehyde to accumulate in your blood faster, so you get your hangover—literally feeling headachy and nauseated—while you're drinking instead of the morning after. The trick is to take one or two capsules of dried kudzu with your first drink.

The advantage here, of course, is that as you start feeling lousy, you'll cut back on your drinking. Acetaldehyde accumulation makes drinking less pleasant and helps keep you from imbibing to excess. The Chinese use kudzu roots or flowers for this purpose.

You can also take kudzu as a tea the morning after, and experts say it can help provide some relief.

Headache

Everyone gets a headache now and then, but an estimated 15 percent of the population—some 40 million Americans—have at least one a week. There's a lot of pain out there.

An estimated 90 percent of headaches are tension headaches, which begin in the back of the neck or head and spread outward with a dull, nonthrobbing pain.

The other 10 percent, including migraines, cluster headaches and caffeine-withdrawal headaches, are caused by the opening and closing (dilation and constriction) of blood vessels in the head that set off pain nerves. Classic migraine is a severe and throbbing headache, usually on one side of the head and often preceded by visual disturbances. Nausea and vomiting often accompany the migraine.

Migraine headaches inflict misery on 25 million Americans. For unknown reasons, about three times as many women as men experience this painful condition. Women often develop migraines just prior to menstrual periods or during pregnancy, and the migraines disappear after menopause in about three-quarters of women.

No single natural therapy—or pharmaceutical, for that matter—works for every type of headache. There are, however, several herbs that can help relieve the different types.

★★★ **Keep pain at bay.** Bay contains compounds known as parthenolides that are extremely useful in preventing migraine. Although the mechanism of these headaches is not thoroughly understood, it appears that release of the neurotransmitter serotonin from blood cells known as platelets plays a causative role. Parthenolides inhibit serotonin release from platelets.

If I had frequent migraines, I might add bay leaves to feverfew, my top-choice herb for treating this condition.

★★★ **Minimize migraines with feverfew.** In my own experience, and this is reflected in the medical literature, feverfew works for about two-thirds of those who use it consistently. Studies published in the *British Medical Journal* agree that taking feverfew regularly prevents migraine attacks. And according to the *Harvard Medical School Health Letter*, "Eating feverfew leaves has become a popular method for preventing migraine attacks in England. Some people for whom conventional treatments for migraine have not worked have turned to feverfew with good results." It's nice to know that I'm in such good company on this one.

People who use feverfew often use fresh leaves, typically ingesting one to four leaves a day to prevent migraines. If you have access to the fresh herb, you might try this approach, but don't expect the leaves to taste good. And some 10 to 18 percent of the people who use fresh feverfew develop mouth sores and/or inflammation of the mouth and tongue.

The good news is that you don't have to eat the leaves to get the full benefits of this herb. You may be able to avoid the side effects by making a tea with about two to eight fresh leaves. Steep them in boiling water, but do not boil them, as boiling may break down the parthenolides.

You can also take this herb in capsules, which is really the easiest way to do it. Depending on the potency of the herb, doses may vary from one capsule a day (60 milligrams) to six capsules a day (about 380 milligrams) of fresh, powdered leaf or two daily 25-milligram capsules of freeze-dried leaf. Feverfew capsules are sold at many herb shops and health food stores. By all means discuss the herb with your doctor if you have a hard time arriving at an appropriate dose.

One caveat: Pregnant women should not take feverfew because of a remote possibility that it might trigger miscarriage. And women who are nursing should not use it because of the possibility of passing the herb to infants in breast milk. Finally, long-term users often report a mild tranquilizing or sedative effect, which may be welcome or unwelcome, depending on your temperament.

★★★ **Ease headache with herbal aspirin.** Commission E, the group of experts that advises the German government about herbs, endorses willow bark as an effective pain reliever for headache and anything else treated by willow's pharmaceutical derivative, aspirin.

When herbalists talk about willow bark as herbal aspirin, they usually mention white willow (*Salix alba*). But this species is rather low in salicin, the aspirin-like chemical in the bark that relieves pain. If you want more headache relief per cup of tea, there are other willow species that are more potent: *S. daphnoides*, *S. fragilis* and *S. purpurea*.

Commission E recommends getting 60 to 120 milligrams of salicin to treat a headache, which works out to 1 teaspoon of the high-salicin barks or 1 to 1½ teaspoons of white willow. More than 86 percent of the salicin in willow is absorbed by the digestive tract, providing a good blood level of the chemical for several hours.

If you're allergic to aspirin, you probably shouldn't take aspirin-like herbs, either. And you should be aware that if aspirin upsets your stomach, willow bark may do the same. Then again, it might not. Leon Chaitow, a British naturopath and osteopath, says, "Unlike aspirin, which is an isolated, concentrated chemical, willow bark acts gently and without aspirin's potential for irritating the stomach." Also, do not give either aspirin or its natural herbal alternatives to children who have headaches with viral infections such as colds or flu, as there's a chance that they might develop Reye's syndrome, a potentially fatal condition that damages the liver and brain.

Heartburn

Heartburn is very common. An estimated 30 percent of adults experience it at least once a month. Diet and lifestyle often contribute to it.

Heartburn develops when the muscular opening from the esophagus into the stomach doesn't work properly. This set of muscles—the lower esophageal sphincter (LES)—opens to allow food into the stomach but then closes to keep stomach acids from washing up into the esophagus. In heartburn, the LES doesn't close completely, and the burning feeling in the chest is actually acid burning the esophagus.

Heartburn is more likely to develop when you eat hurriedly, on the run, standing up or wolfing down your food without chewing it thoroughly. Fried foods, saturated fats, sugar, alcohol, cigarettes and coffee have all been associated with heartburn. To help prevent it, try to have meals and snacks when you're relaxed instead of on the go. It also helps to have a diet of fruits, vegetables and whole grains.

In addition to avoiding aggravating foods and eating habits, here are some herbs that can help.

★★ **Douse the burn with angelica.** Aromatherapists wisely suggest oil of angelica as useful for heartburn in adults and colic and gas in children. Angelica is a member of the carrot family, and many members of that plant family seem to have a soothing action on the digestive tract, a quality that herbalists call carminative.

If you have heartburn frequently, you should discuss it with your doctor. You might also wish to indulge in my Angelade, which contains six relatives of angelica, all carminative. You'll need a juicer to make this one, as Angelade consists of juiced angelica stalks, carrots, celery, fennel, garlic, parsley and parsnips. (You may have to add some water and spices to make it drinkable.)

If you don't have access to fresh angelica, it's okay to leave it out and go with just the other ingredients. In fact, it doesn't really make any difference how much of each you use. Simply pick your favorites, then mix and match until you create a juice that tickles your fancy.

★★ **Cool the fire with camomile.** Joe and Terry Graedon, co-authors of *The People's Pharmacy* and *Graedon's Best Medicine*, share my opinion that camomile is the first-choice herb for heartburn and stomach distress.

★★ **Reduce acid with licorice.** I agree with Michael Murray, N.D., co-author of *Encyclopedia of Natural Medicine* and several other scholarly books on nutritional and naturopathic healing, that deglycyrrhizinated licorice (DGL) successfully treats both heartburn and ulcers of the stomach and esophagus. Many studies show that licorice is an antispasmodic and that it reduces production of stomach acid, thereby decreasing heartburn.

The caveat is that while licorice and its extracts are safe for normal use in moderate amounts (up to about three cups of tea a day) long-term use (more than six weeks) or ingestion of larger amounts can produce headache, lethargy, sodium and water retention, excessive loss of potassium and high blood pressure. A cup of licorice tea now and then to relieve heartburn is safe.

Hemorrhoids

Estimates vary, but it looks like hemorrhoids affect one-third of Americans— some 75 million people. All four people in my family have experienced them, more often when we get away from the high-fiber diet that we eat at home.

Hemorrhoids are varicose veins of the anus. Anal veins drain blood away from the area. They expand (dilate) during defecation and shrink back to normal size afterward. However, repeated straining during defecation, which is a common result of constipation, can interfere with the normal functioning of these veins. They may become permanently swollen, causing pain and itching.

The best way to deal with hemorrhoids is to prevent them, and the best way to do that is to prevent constipation. You'll find several herbs that are good for relieving chronic constipation mentioned in this chapter. (For additional details, see page 44.)

Basically, staying regular boils down to eating a high-fiber diet, with lots of fruits and vegetables, and drinking plenty of nonalcoholic fluids. I daresay that anyone who regularly eats five fibrous fruits and five fibrous veggies a day will not suffer from constipation. In other words, a preventive ounce of carrots or apples—and of course, prunes—is worth a pound of buckthorn, an herbal laxative, taken later.

If you develop hemorrhoids, here are some herbs to try.

★★ **Comfort your bottom with comfrey.** Comfrey is rich in allantoin, a wound-healing chemical that is anti-inflammatory, stimulates the immune system and hastens the formation of new skin. You can moisten powdered comfrey with vegetable oil and apply the paste. Or you can pound the leaf to soften the fuzzy hairs it's covered with and apply the leaf itself, topically. You don't have to worry about washing it off, as the residue will come off the next time you shower.

★★ **Put on a plantain poultice.** Plantain has a strong folk reputation as a hemorrhoid remedy. This herb contains allantoin, the same soothing compound found in comfrey. If I were caught in the bush with a hemorrhoid and without my Tucks, I'd create a poultice and apply it to the afflicted area.

★★ **Prevent constipation with psyllium.** In one study, 51 people with hemorrhoids received a psyllium preparation. More than three-quarters (84 percent) reported improvement—less pain, itching, bleeding and discomfort on defecation. Commission E, the German herbal advisory panel, recommends taking anywhere from four to ten teaspoons of psyllium seeds a day for constipation. It's easy to get that much by using a commercial product such as Metamucil, which is made with psyllium seeds. Simply follow the directions on the package.

Psyllium works by absorbing water in the gut and swelling considerably, which adds bulk to stool and triggers the muscle contractions we experience as "the urge." If you use psyllium, make sure you drink enough fluids. You should get at least eight (eight-ounce) glasses of water or juice a day. And watch how you react to this herb if you have allergies. If allergic symptoms develop after you take it once, don't use it again.

★★ **Shrink hemorrhoids with witch hazel.** For a long time, I thought the *H* in Preparation H stood for *Hamamelis*. This is the Latin name for witch hazel, the active ingredient in the popular Preparation H Cleansing Pads. (I guess I should have guessed that the *H* actually stands for hemorrhoids.) Witch hazel is also the active ingredient in Tucks, the commercial pharmaceutical product often recommended for hemorrhoids.

Witch hazel is a soothing, cooling astringent that can help relieve hemorrhoidal pain and itching. But you really don't have to spend extra for a brand name. Simply make a compress using witch hazel, which is available at pharmacies for a much lower price. Just tuck a fresh compress in place whenever you feel the need for a little soothing. Then forget it's there and go about your business.

High Blood Pressure

High blood pressure, or hypertension, is generally defined as a blood pressure greater than 140/90. The first number (systolic) is the force that blood exerts on the artery walls when the heart is pumping. The second number (diastolic) is the residual force that remains when the heart relaxes between beats. Any blood pressure reading below "high"—say, a borderline 138/88—is safer, but you should still try getting it down closer to what's considered normal, 120/80. That's because any elevation in blood pressure raises your risk for heart attack and stroke.

About 50 million Americans have high blood pressure, which is often called the silent killer. While the condition itself causes no symptoms, it sets the stage for a heart attack or stroke. In the past few decades, doctors and other health professionals have made a big push to detect high blood pressure and treat it more aggressively, and the rate of heart attack has indeed gone down. But the problem, in my opinion, is that doctors are too quick to treat this condition with synthetic drugs. About half of the people diagnosed with high blood pressure have borderline to mildly high blood pressure. There's plenty of solid evidence that for them, diet and lifestyle changes, including regular exercise, stress management and self-monitoring with a home blood pressure device, work just as well as drugs, with no side effects.

Diet and lifestyle modifications all tend to provide a sense of control that in itself may be beneficial. But don't expect the pharmaceutical industry to encourage the natural way. It would cut into the $2.5 billion-a-year market for antihypertensive medication.

There are a number of herbs that can help control blood pressure.

★★★ **To chip away points, crunch on celery.** Celery has long been recommended in traditional Chinese medicine for lowering high blood pressure, and experimental evidence bears this out. In one study, injecting laboratory animals with celery extract significantly lowered their blood pressure. In humans, eating as few as four celery stalks has done the same.

★★★ **Enjoy garlic in copious quantities.** This wonder herb not only helps normalize blood pressure, it also reduces cholesterol. In a scientifically rigorous study, people with high blood pressure were given about one clove of garlic a day for 12 weeks. Afterward they exhibited significantly lower diastolic blood pressure and cholesterol levels.

"We now know that garlic can reduce hypertension, even in quantities as small as a half-ounce per week," says Varro Tyler, Ph.D., dean and professor emeritus of pharmacognosy (natural product pharmacy) at Purdue University in West Lafayette, Indiana. A half-ounce per week works out to about one clove a day. If you cook with garlic and use it in your salads, getting that much should be a snap. If you haven't yet developed a taste for it, you can take garlic in capsule form. With so many health benefits associated with this herb, I'd recommend finding many ways to enjoy it in your food.

★★ **Help your heart with hawthorn.** Hawthorn extract can widen (dilate) blood vessels, especially the coronary arteries, according to a report published in the *Lawrence Review of Natural Products*, a respected newsletter. Hawthorn has been used as a heart tonic for centuries.

If you'd like to try this powerful heart medicine, discuss it with your doctor. You can try a tea made with one teaspoon of dried herb per cup of boiling water and drink up to two cups a day.

High Cholesterol

The total cholesterol level of the average American is higher than 200 milligrams per deciliter (mg/dl) of blood. Because heart attack risk rises sharply above that level, the American Heart Association urges everyone to take measures to reduce cholesterol if it's anywhere near that high.

How far below 200 should you go to feel that your risk is significantly less? That's not entirely clear, but research suggests that very low cholesterol levels, below 150 or so, increase risk of death from other causes, including liver cancer, lung disease and certain kinds of stroke. My reaction is that people should strive for a cholesterol range of 170 to 190.

To make matters more complicated, there are two kinds of cholesterol—low-density lipoproteins (LDL), which increase risk of heart attack, and high-density lipoproteins (HDL), which actually reduce it. You want to get your total cholesterol down below 190. But if you have high cholesterol, your doctor may focus specifically on your LDL levels and have you work to reduce those, since the "bad" kind is most clearly linked to heart disease.

Any and probably all plant fibers can lower cholesterol. That means eating a diet that includes lots of fruits, vegetables and whole grains, hopefully one with a minimum of fats.

Along with getting adequate fiber from the foods you eat, there are a number of individual foods and herbs that can prove helpful. Here are a few of my favorites.

★★★ **Pare down your cholesterol with pectin.** Scottish studies showed that over a period of three weeks, a daily snack of two carrots lowered cholesterol levels by 10 to 20 percent in study participants. Carrots are high in the fiber pectin. Other good sources of pectin include apples and the white inner layer of citrus rinds. Enjoy these foods on a daily basis. (Yes, if you're eating an orange, nibble on a little of the white stuff.)

I know that juicing is really big these days, so I'd like to offer a little advice. If you want to take these fruits and vegetables in beverage form, fine. But don't use a juicer on them if you want to get the full benefit of their pectin content. Just whir them in a blender instead. If you use a juicer, you extract most of the fiber, and only about 10 percent of the cholesterol-lowering pectin remains.

You can also take supplements. University of Florida scientists reported that three tablespoons of grapefruit pectin daily, taken in capsules or as a food additive, can lower cholesterol by about 8 percent. If you go the supplement route, however, you should be aware that this type of fiber interferes with the uptake of certain important nutrients, including beta-carotene, boron, calcium, copper, iron and zinc. This is less of a problem when you consume the whole plant, because the plant itself supplies extra nutrients. But if you take pectin capsules, remember to eat your fruits and vegetables at a later meal to make sure you don't trigger any deficiencies.

★★ **Take advantage of avocado.** Avocado is one of the highest-fat fruits, so people with heart disease often avoid it. But according to a report in the *Lawrence Review of Natural Products*, a respected newsletter, avocado can help reduce cholesterol. In one study, women were given a choice of a diet high in monounsaturated fats (olive oil) with avocado or a diet rich in complex carbohydrates (starches and sugars.) After six weeks, those on the olive oil-avocado diet showed an 8.2 percent reduction in cholesterol.

I'm not advocating that you should cut back on complex carbohydrates, which are important to a healthy diet, but I am suggesting that you enjoy an occasional avocado. It contains some unique chemicals that you may not be getting elsewhere.

★★ **Bring on the beans.** Beans are high in fiber and low in fat—just the ticket for lowering cholesterol. And they contain lecithin, a nutrient that also helps cut cholesterol. One study showed that a cup and a half of dried lentils or kidney beans a day, about the amount in a bowl of bean soup, can lower total cholesterol levels by 19 percent.

Hives

Hives are itchy red skin welts with whitish centers. Medically, they're known as urticaria or nettle rash, a name inspired by the fact that the stinging nettle plant can cause them.

Hives are a reaction to histamine, a substance secreted by special cells known as mast cells that are distributed throughout the body. Small amounts of histamine, incidentally, are also injected into you when you bump up against the tiny hairs that cover the stinging nettle plant.

The histamine made by your body plays a role in producing the symptoms of hay fever–type allergies, including sneezing and watery eyes. That's why *anti*histamines, substances that block the natural action of histamines, can help to treat so many allergy symptoms, including hives.

Some 15 to 20 percent of Americans experience hives at some point in their lives, most frequently as young adults.

Just about anything that can cause an allergic reaction can cause hives, including certain foods, aspirin and many other drugs. Sometimes unexpected things cause hives; about 3 percent of people who use sunscreen get hives, for example. But in many cases, the cause of hives remains a mystery.

Prescription and over-the-counter antihistamines are the standard medical treatment for hives. There are also a number of herbal approaches.

★★★ **Befriend a gem of an herb.** Jewelweed is one of my favorite herbs for hives. It contains a compound called lawsone that works wonders.

I learned about lawsone's anti-hive action at the 1995 Annual Spring Wildflower Outing in Wintergreen, Virginia. My long-time friend, herbalist Jim Troy, slapped both of my wrists with nettle plant until both stung mightily. I had with me a bottled solution of lawsone which Robert Rosen, Ph.D., a chemist at Rutgers University in New Brunswick, New Jersey, had provided. I rubbed the solution onto my right wrist and enjoyed instant relief. The hives on my left wrist kept right on itching. This mini-experiment convinced me that any plant containing the compound lawsone, such as jewelweed, is worth considering as a treatment for hives.

If you'd like to try this remedy, you'll have to have access to fresh jewelweed, which is fairly common throughout the country. If you aren't sure what jewelweed looks like, you should find someone in your area who can show you the plant—a local herbalist, perhaps, or an agricultural extension agent.

★★★ **Heal hives with stinging nettle.** Yes, I'm talking about the very same plant that will produce a welt if its hairs inject their histamine into you. Andrew

Weil, M.D., an herb advocate who teaches at the University of Arizona College of Medicine in Tucson and author of *Natural Health, Natural Medicine*, suggests using freeze–dried nettle leaf extract to treat hives and allergies. This might sound illogical, but the plant apparently doesn't contain enough histamine to be a problem when it's taken orally, and it does contain substances that help heal hives.

Stinging nettle is sold in capsules in health food stores. Dr. Weil suggests taking one or two every two to four hours, as needed.

★★ **Prevent allergic reactions with parsley.** One scientific study showed that parsley inhibits the secretion of histamine. If you have hives, try juicing some parsley and adding it to some other vegetable juice, such as carrot or tomato, to make it more palatable.

Indigestion

What most people refer to as a stomachache often has nothing to do with the stomach. The discomfort can emanate from any of several digestive organs—hence the name *indigestion*.

Indigestion can have any number of causes—some quite minor, some quite serious. For this reason, many doctors recommend that people with chronic, re-current, or severe indigestion get examined to rule out any underlyling health problems.

For ordinary, everyday indigestion, there are hundreds of herbs that can help. Here are several that I recommend.

★★★ **Calm a grumpy gut with camomile.** Commission E, the German group of scientists that makes recommendations on herbal safety and effective-ness, considers camomile effective for relieving many gastrointestinal complaints, including indigestion. Andrew Weil, M.D., professor at the University of Arizona College of Medicine in Tucson and author of *Natural Health, Natural Medicine*, says that the best home remedies for upset stomach are camomile and pepper-mint tea. Personally, I prefer peppermint, but both are effective.

While drinking camomile tea is fine, the tincture is probably more effective. Camomile tea has only 10 to 15 percent of the herb's carminative essential oil, while tinctures prepared with 100-proof alcohol have much more.

★★★ **Be partial to peppermint.** Most herbalists, myself included, have a spe-cial regard for peppermint's ability to relieve indigestion. I've needed peppermint more often since 1990, when the Food and Drug Administration (FDA) gave me a bad case of indigestion by ruling that peppermint is ineffective for stomach distress. This does not mean that peppermint is useless. Frankly, it means that the FDA's evaluation was useless.

Commission E endorses peppermint tea for treating indigestion. Given a choice between an FDA pronouncement and a Commission E endorsement, I'd go for the German decision. Those folks did some research and really know what they're about.

Peppermint tea works well, but being a native son of Alabama, I'm also partial to mint juleps, which, it turns out, work even better. Varro Tyler, Ph.D., dean and professor emeritus of pharmacognosy (natural product pharmacy) at Purdue University in West Lafayette, Indiana, notes that most of the carminative oils in peppermint and other mints are relatively insoluble in water. As a result, mint tea doesn't contain much of the plant's stomach-soothing constituents. It does contain enough to make it effective, but a peppermint tincture, which is made with alcohol, contains more. So if for some reason you don't want to drink a julep, you can use a tincture instead. Follow the package directions.

★★ **Allay distress with angelica.** Angelica root is good for treating indigestion, mild stomach cramps and lack of appetite, according to Commission E. The suggested daily dose is a tea made with two to three teaspoons of dried herb per cup of boiling water, or up to one teaspoon of tincture.

Infertility

Infertility is generally defined as an inability to conceive after six months to one year of trying. An estimated 20 percent of couples have trouble conceiving. Rising maternal age is a factor; as women are having babies later in life, the risk of infertility rises. Among men, falling sperm counts may also be part of the problem.

Treating infertility has become a huge medical industry during the past few decades, with doctors doing everything from prescribing fertility drugs to arranging for test-tube babies (in vitro fertilization). These well-publicized procedures can cost up to $10,000 apiece.

While some infertility problems in women can be addressed by having children earlier, men need to try some tactics to raise their sperm counts. The following section highlights primarily the natural alternatives that can be helpful for men.

Infertility is a major heartache, and it may require going the high-tech route.

But before you try a high-tech solution, you'll want to thoroughly explore possible causes with your doctor to find out whether there are lifestyle or other changes that you can make to improve your chances of conception. And while you're at it, consider some natural alternatives.

★★ **Build your meals around foods rich in B$_6$.** People who advocate micronutrient supplementation often recommend vitamin B$_6$ for infertility. The best sources of this nutrient, in descending order of potency, are cauliflower, watercress, spinach, garden cress, bananas, okra, onions, broccoli, squash, kale, kohlrabi, brussels sprouts, peas and radishes.

★★ **Stimulate sperm with ginger.** According to reports of research with animals in Saudi Arabia, ginger significantly increased sperm count and motility. I hesitate to extrapolate one animal study to humans, but ginger is so safe and tasty that if I were troubled by a low sperm count or poor sperm motility, I wouldn't hesitate to reach for ginger tea, ginger ale, gingerbread and dishes spiced with this tangy herb.

★★ **Enhance potency with ginseng.** California herbalist Kathi Keville, author of *The Illustrated Herb Encyclopedia* and *Herbs for Health and Healing*, tells two stories of infertile men who started taking ginseng, schisandra and saw palmetto to build up their physical stamina. Some time later, both of their wives became pregnant.

While I wouldn't hang my hat on this anecdote, ginseng has been revered in Asia for centuries as a male potency and longevity tonic. There is some research with animals suggesting that ginseng stimulates sexual activity, and of course, you need that to conceive.

Inhibited Sexual Desire in Women

Anyone, man or woman, can lose interest in sex. In women, the condition used to be called frigidity, but sex therapists have dropped that judgmental term in favor of the more neutral terms *loss of libido* or *inhibited sexual desire*.

Many factors can cause loss of desire, including illness, injury, emotional stress (especially because a relationship is on the rocks), alcohol and many prescription medications, particularly antidepressants. I suggest that before you go to a psychotherapist or write yourself off as asexual, make a list of all the medications that you take, both prescription and over-the-counter. Then take the list to your doctor or pharmacist and ask if any of these medications have side effects that could be affecting your sex life. If so, ask your doctor if you can substitute other medications that might have a less dastardly effect.

Once you've ruled out common causes of libido loss, then you might try some herbal approaches.

★★ **Use Chinese angelica as an aphrodisiac.** The Chinese say that this herb, also known as *dang gui*, does for women what ginseng does for men—it's an all-purpose sexual and reproductive tonic.

Because of its reputation as a sex enhancer, Chinese angelica is one of the most widely used herbs in Chinese women's medicine. Typically, three to six teaspoons of powdered root are added to a pint of boiling water. Women drink up to three cups of the tea a day. (Do not take this herb if you are pregnant, however.)

★★ **Restore desire with ginseng.** Even though ginseng has long been considered an aphrodisiac for men, I've read reports of women who felt greater sexual responsiveness after consuming it.

Nowadays, several herbalists I know suggest ginseng for loss of sexual desire in women. This herb is very expensive, so few people take very much. The typical dose is a half-teaspoon or so of tincture in juice.

★ **Build interest with anise.** Anise is high in anethole, a compound with effects similar to those of the female sex hormone estrogen. It has a folk reputation for increasing milk secretion, promoting menstruation, facilitating childbirth and increasing libido in women. Some scientists say that estrogen has nothing to do with sex drive, but I believe that plant estrogens (phytoestrogens) enhance lust for life—and plain old lust as well.

Insect Bites and Stings

Doctors generally recommend pain relievers, ice packs and meat tenderizer to treat insect bites and stings. (Applying a dab of commercial meat tenderizer directly to a sting neutralizes venom.) These are all reasonable approaches. There are also a number of good herbal alternatives.

★★ **End pain with calendula.** I'm a fan of Maude Grieve, whose *Modern Herbal*, written in 1931, is now a classic in the field. Grieve writes picturesquely that calendula flower "rubbed on the affected part, is an admirable remedy for the pain and swelling caused by the sting of a wasp or bee." I believe her, and I would try it if I were stung and had some fresh calendula close at hand.

★★ **Apply a garlic and onion poultice.** Both garlic and onions contain enzymes that break down chemical substances known as prostaglandins that the body releases in response to pain.

Interestingly enough, garlic and onions work both internally and externally. You can make a poultice of these herbs and apply them directly to insect bites and stings. You can also get a measure of relief by eating foods that contain them.

One further note: Onion skin is an extremely good source of the anti-allergic chemical quercetin, which is especially good for relieving inflammation. You can get the added benefit of quercetin by leaving the skin on when you cook soups or stews. Fish out the skin just before serving; it will have released a good amount of quercetin into the dish, along with a rich, brown color.

★★ **Pick fresh plantain.** Wherever I go—from the Appalachians to the Andes to the Rockies—plantain is one of the first herbs my botanical friends mention for bug bite. It's the first thing I apply at home, too, since it is a common weed in my lawn. (You need to rub on the fresh herb for this remedy to work.)

Edward E. Shook, author of *Advanced Treatise on Herbology*, tells a story about a woman who got a bee sting on her hand, and her entire arm began to swell. He told her to wash plantain leaves, make a poultice and apply it to the sting. The next day the woman returned, healed. I didn't see this happen, but I do know that plantain is many herbalists' herb of choice for bee stings.

Insomnia

Insomnia is a broad term that encompasses any and all difficulties with sleep, including the inability to fall asleep or to stay asleep.

We live in a country that has a hard time getting enough sleep. About a third of Americans experience insomnia regularly, and up to ten million rely on sedative prescriptions to help them fall asleep. That's a whole lot of sleeping pills.

Pharmaceutical sedatives work, but they can become addictive, and they interfere with natural sleep cycles. You won't be surprised to learn that I prefer natural alternatives, of which there are several.

★★★ **Let lemon balm lull you to sleep.** Also known as melissa, lemon balm is endorsed as both a sedative and stomach soother by Commission E, the body of scientists that advises the German government about herb safety and effectiveness. The sedative action is attributed largely to a group of chemicals in the plant called terpenes. Several other herbs—juniper, ginger, basil and clove—are better endowed with some of these chemicals, but none of them has the combination that lemon balm contains, and none of them has its reputation as a bedtime herb.

I suggest trying a tea made with two to four teaspoons of dried herb per cup of boiling water.

★★★ **Sip valerian tea, catch some Zzz's.** Drinking a tea made with one to two teaspoons of dried valerian root shortly before bedtime will promote sleepiness, according to Commission E. In fact, the commission considers the tea so safe that it also endorses drinking it up to several times a day to relieve restlessness, anxiety and nervousness.

Valerian has a fairly rank aroma and taste. If its earthiness is not to your liking, you can always opt for a tincture or capsules instead.

Unlike prescription sleep or anxiety medications, valerian is not considered habit-forming, nor does it produce a "hangover," as do medications in the Valium group.

Some naturopaths I respect suggest that you treat insomnia by drinking valerian root tea about 30 minutes before retiring. Others suggest taking 150 to 300 milligrams of a standardized extract (0.8 percent valeric acid).

★★ **Ensure slumber with lavender.** It's nice to see lavender approved by Commission E for insomnia. I've seen accounts of British hospitals using lavender oil to help patients sleep at night. The hospitals administer the oil either in a warm bath or sprinkled onto bedclothes.

Lavender oil is also a favorite of aromatherapists, who use it for all sorts of ailments, including insomnia. Some components of lavender oil affect cell membranes, interrupting the interaction of cells with each other. Because the oil helps to slow nerve impulses, it can help reduce irritability and bring on sleep. It also has an anesthetic effect.

Laryngitis

Laryngitis is an inflammation of the vocal cords that causes hoarseness or voice loss and usually a dry, sore throat. More and more these days at pharmacies and health food stores, you can find herbal lozenges for sore throat and laryngitis. They taste pretty good. If you have chronic laryngitis, though, see your doctor: It may be a symptom of a serious condition. But for an occasional bout of laryngitis, you can turn to herbs for help. Here are several good ones to try.

★★★ **Choose herbs containing cineole.** Cineole is an expectorant that can help bring relief. Here are several herbs with high cineole content, in descending order of potency: cardamom, eucalyptus, spearmint, rosemary, sweet Annie, ginger, nutmeg, lavender, bee balm, peppermint and tansy. I suggest making a tea using a selection of these herbs, and go heavy on the ginger. Add some pineapple juice before drinking.

★★ **Soothe your throat with horehound.** This herb has been used for centuries to treat coughs and other respiratory problems like laryngitis. Commission E, the body of experts that advises the German government about herbs, endorses horehound for bronchial problems, including laryngitis. The suggested dosage is a tea made with one to two teaspoons of dried herb per cup of boiling water.

But wouldn't you know that the Food and Drug Administration declared horehound ineffective in treating sore throat and laryngitis? The problem is not with horehound but rather with the agency charged with protecting and promoting the public health. Horehound is one of the first herbs I suggest for throat problems. I'd recommend a strong horehound tea with lemon, licorice and stevia, which is available in many health food stores. You can open a tea bag and add a pinch of herb in place of artificial sweetener.

★★ **Minimize discomfort with the mallows.** The mallows, including marsh mallow, the herbal forerunner of our pillowy candy treat, have been used for thousands of years as throat soothers. They are useful in treating laryngitis, colds, coughs, sore throat and bronchitis.

Mallows contain a special gelatinous fiber, mucilage, that soothes mucous membranes and helps protect them from bacteria and inflammation. Commission E approves mallows for throat pain, inflammation and irritation. Sounds like a laryngitis treatment to me.

Macular Degeneration

Macular degeneration affects more than 25 percent of Americans over 65 years old. It is the leading cause of blindness in the elderly. You're at somewhat greater risk of having macular degeneration if you are farsighted or smoke cigarettes. People with light-colored eyes and a family history of the condition are also at greater risk.

I can't guarantee that if you eat your veggies you'll have good vision when you're as old as Methuselah. But if the studies I've reviewed are correct, you'll certainly have better vision than you would if you ate junk food instead.

Here's why: There is some indication that cell damage caused by highly reactive oxygen molecules (free radicals) plays a role in an eye condition known as macular degeneration. Antioxidants are substances that neutralize these free radicals and prevent them from doing harm. And fruits and vegetables, especially leafy vegetables, are simply your best sources of these beneficial substances.

The macula is the central and most sensitive portion of the retina, the nerve-rich area in the back of the eye that is necessary for sight. For unknown reasons, after around age 60, the macula begins to break down. As it degenerates, central vision and fine detail perception deteriorate. (Peripheral vision remains unaffected.)

Conventional medical therapies don't help much with macular degeneration, which makes nutritional approaches look all the more appealing. Quite a few foods and herbs might help.

★★★ **Sharpen your vision with fruit.** Bilberry and its relatives, blueberry, cranberry, huckleberry, blackberry, grape, plum and wild cherry, have been used traditionally for problems with visual acuity. And scientific research has validated this folk medicine approach.

All of these fruits contain compounds known as anthocyanosides, which are potent antioxidants. In one study, daily treatment with 400 milligrams of bilberry and 20 milligrams of the famous antioxidant beta-carotene improved many participants' night vision and enlarged their visual fields. Bilberry anthocyanosides also strengthen the capillaries in the retina, which helps slow macular degeneration.

★★ **Become a fan of greens.** One study, done by ophthalmologist Johanna Seddon, M.D., of the Massachusetts Eye and Ear Infirmary in Boston, involved surveying almost 900 people, 326 of whom had macular degeneration. Dr. Seddon found that eating antioxidant-rich fruits and vegetables at least five times a week cut the risk of macular degeneration in half.

Collard greens, the popular soul food, and spinach, Popeye's favorite food, stood out in Dr. Seddon's study. These vegetables contain the beneficial compounds lutein and zeaxanthin. Vegetables that contain similar compounds that may provide eye protection include bok choy, broccoli, brussels sprouts, cabbage, kale, kohlrabi, mustard greens, radishes, turnip greens and watercress.

Dr. Seddon's study also found that taking vitamin C and E supplements didn't do much to help prevent macular degeneration, even though both are potent antioxidants. This strengthens my ongoing argument that you're better off with whole, nutrient-rich foods and herbs rather than single-nutrient supplements.

★★ **Nourish your eyes with ginkgo.** Ginkgo extracts help maintain good blood flow to the retina. In one six-month study, people who received 80 milligrams of a standardized ginkgo extract twice daily significantly improved their long-distance vision. Another study suggests that ginkgo extract may even reverse damage in the retina. To me this suggests that you should try mixing ginkgo with antioxidant mint teas.

Ginkgo leaves actually contain very little of the active compounds. The best way to get the full benefits of this herb is to use a standardized extract—a 50:1 preparation, which means that 50 pounds of leaves have been processed to make 1 pound of extract. (I occasionally add a few leaves to my blended fresh fruit juices anyway.) The suggested dose of standardized extract is 150 to 300 milligrams a day. (In amounts higher than 240 milligrams, ginkgo may cause diarrhea, irritability and restlessness, so if you experience any of these symptoms, opt for a lower dose.)

Menopause

Menopause means the cessation of menstruation. Most women experience menopause during their late forties and early fifties. Sometimes it happens quickly. More frequently, it takes a few years for menstrual periods to cease.

As menopause develops, estrogen production declines, often causing one or more discomforts: anxiety, breast tenderness, depression, dry skin, headache, hot flashes, incontinence, insomnia, irritability, nervousness, night sweats and vaginal dryness.

Of this list, hot flashes are most common, affecting about 85 percent of menopausal women. Hot flashes usually occur without warning, but some women notice that emotional stress, exercise, alcohol and certain foods may trigger them.

Hot flashes and other menopausal symptoms are rare in vegetarian cultures, especially among people who consume a lot of legumes, like black beans, mung beans and soybeans.

Why? Because beans and many other plants have mild estrogenic activity, thanks to phytoestrogens. These compounds include isoflavones, lignans, phytosterols and saponins.

Phytoestrogens are weaker than the body's own estrogen. In premenopausal women, phytoestrogens compete with women's own, more potent estrogen, reducing the total effects of estrogen. But as women's estrogen production falls, phytoestrogens supplement this hormone.

Put another way, when women have too much biological estrogen, phytoestrogens lower the burden; when they have too little, phytoestrogens pinch-hit.

In addition to a high-phytoestrogen vegetarian diet, a number of specific herbs can help relieve many symptoms associated with menopause. Here's my selection.

★★ Cool hot flashes with black cohosh. Long recommended for "female complaints," this herb contains estrogenic substances that help relieve menopause discomforts, especially hot flashes. In one study of 110 menopausal women, half were given black cohosh root extract, while the other half took an inactive preparation (a placebo). After eight weeks, blood tests showed significant estrogenic activity in the women taking the herb.

In another study, women with vaginal dryness due to menopause experienced similar relief whether taking black cohosh or pharmaceutical estrogen.

★★ Elevate estrogen with licorice. Licorice contains natural estrogenic compounds. Like the isoflavones in soy, glycyrrhizin, the active ingredient in licorice, appears to reduce estrogen levels in women when they're too high and increase the levels when they're too low.

Could licorice candy help women with menopausal discomforts? Possibly, but read the label. Most American licorice contains extracts of licorice plus anise, which contains a chemical (anethole) that is less estrogenic than glycyrrhizin. Many health food stores carry candies made from pure licorice.

Licorice and its extracts are safe for normal use in moderate amounts, but long-term use or ingestion of larger amounts can produce headache, lethargy, sodium and water retention, excessive loss of potassium and high blood pressure. A safe daily dose of a true licorice confection is said to be five grams, or less than a quarter-ounce. It's hard to stop when something tastes that good, but you'll just have to control yourself.

★ Drown discomforts in alfalfa tea. Alfalfa has demonstrable estrogenic activity. The leaves make a pleasant-tasting tea. If you have lupus or a family history of lupus, however, steer clear of alfalfa sprouts. There's some evidence that they may trigger lupus in sensitive individuals.

Menstrual Cramps

Women who think menstrual cramps are no big deal haven't experienced a full-blown case of these painful spasms. They can feel like a charley horse in your abdomen, and they may be accompanied by diarrhea and nausea.

If you experience really intense menstrual pain, doctors recommend getting a check-up to make sure that your cramps aren't brought on by an underlying medical problem such as endometriosis or a pelvic infection. Once your doctor rules out other causes, try one of these herbs to help ease your monthly cramps.

★★★ Banish cramps with black haw. Under the name crampbark, this herb was recognized as a treatment for menstrual cramps in most pharmacology reference books through the nineteenth century. The bark contains at least four substances that help relax the uterus. Two (aesculetin and scopoletin) also help relieve muscle spasms. With so much folklore and science to recommend it, black haw would be one of the first remedies that I'd suggest to my daughter if she came to me complaining of cramps.

★★★ **Choose an Asian aid.** Also known as *dang gui*, Chinese angelica is one of the most widely used herbs in Chinese traditional medicine. It is considered a female tonic, especially good for menstrual cramps, and is highly recommended by experts in Oriental medicine.

★★★ **Relax with raspberry leaf tea.** Many women herbalists I respect recommend raspberry leaf tea for easing menstrual cramps. One study showed that this herb helps relax the uterus. It's also popular for soothing the uterine irritability associated with pregnancy.

Researchers don't know the active compound in raspberry, but they speculate that it might be Pycnogenol (an oligomeric procyanidin, or OPC). That makes sense to me. In one study, taking 200 milligrams of OPC daily over two cycles eliminated or significantly relieved menstrual cramps and/or premenstrual syndrome in 50 to 60 percent of the women who took them. Among women who took OPCs for four cycles, the number who benefited was even higher— 66 to 80 percent.

You can buy pure OPC in the form of Pycnogenol, but it's an expensive supplement. I'd suggest trying raspberry leaf tea instead.

★★ **Get relief from bilberry.** Bilberry contains chemicals called anthocyanidins, which have muscle-relaxant properties, and it also contains OPCs. For menstrual cramps, some herbalists suggest taking 20 to 40 milligrams of concentrated bilberry extract three times a day. If you can't find extracts, try a half-cup of fresh bilberries or blueberries, which have similar properties.

★★ **Chase pain with chasteberry.** The small fruits of the chasteberry tree have been used for menstrual disorders since Greco-Roman times. I'm convinced that chasteberry is effective.

Motion Sickness

Motion sickness is the combination of nausea, dizziness and I'd-rather-be-dead feelings that many people experience on boats, cars, trains or planes.

Drugstores stock several different motion sickness remedies, most notably the antihistamine dimenhydrinate (Dramamine). Transderm Scōp, a patch that delivers the drug scopolamine through the skin, is a popular treatment, but it can cause side effects that prompt concerns about its safety. It has been known to cause hallucinations and convulsions in some people. And dimenhydrinate can also cause problems, making you drowsy and dopey.

Fortunately, there's one herbal alternative that beats motion sickness drugs every time. I'm talking about ginger. It's not the only effective herbal remedy, but it's certainly the best that I'm aware of.

★★★ **Make ginger your first choice.** Varro Tyler, Ph.D., dean and professor emeritus of pharmacognosy (natural product pharmacy) at Purdue University in West Lafayette, Indiana, endorses ginger: "To prevent motion sickness, swallow two capsules 30 minutes before departure and then one or two more as symptoms begin to occur, probably about every four hours."

I use ginger myself. It works. Sometimes I munch the ginger raw, but chances are that you'd prefer a few teaspoons in tea. You can also buy ginger capsules at health food stores. Or you can simply drink ginger ale, but if you do, make sure the label says that it's made with real ginger. A lot of ginger ale these days is artificially flavored.

Yet another ginger-filled remedy is my Stomach-Settler Tea: Chop up a two-inch section of ginger root and stir it in with dashes of camomile flowers, fennel, orange peel, peppermint and/or spearmint. Steep these with a few cups of water for 15 minutes. (You might also add a dash of cinnamon. Back in King Solomon's time, cinnamon tea was used to prevent nausea. Queen Peggy, Mrs. Duke, still uses it this way.)

If you have a juicer on hand, you might try juiceman Jay Kordich's Ginger Jolt—two apples, one pear and a one-inch section of ginger root. If all you have is a blender, try this Digestive Delight from naturopath Michael Murray, N.D.: one cup of fresh pineapple chunks, one or two kiwifruits, a one-inch section of ginger root and a few pinches of mint.

★ **Give queasiness the raspberries.** Raspberry leaf tea is widely recommended for the nausea of morning sickness. Some herbalists also suggest it for motion sickness. I have no problem with that: Ginger and raspberry tea mix nicely.

Nausea

Nausea, as I'm sure you know, is that horrible abdominal sensation that makes you feel as if you're going to vomit. And vomiting means losing your lunch, plus a good deal of stomach acid as well, which is why it causes a burning sensation in the chest and throat.

Nausea and vomiting can be caused by many things: infections of the digestive tract (gastroenteritis), inner ear disorders, overindulgence in alcohol or foods, intestinal parasites, morning sickness in pregnancy, motion sickness, emotional stress and toxic overloads on the liver.

Frequently, one good upchuck is all it takes to relieve nausea. You just vomit and get it over with. But in other cases, nausea persists even after the stomach has emptied, and you try to vomit without result, a condition known as dry heaves. That's when the herbal remedies in this chapter might help.

★★★ **Calm your gut with ginger.** One study showed that ginger appears to be as effective as the prescription drug metoclopramide (Reglan, Clopra) in reducing the nausea and vomiting caused by cancer chemotherapy. This is one use for ginger that you should discuss with your doctor. If he says that your blood-clotting ability is impaired, you should not take this herb while undergoing chemotherapy.

Of course, ginger helps with nausea from less extreme causes as well. I discuss its anti-nausea benefits at some length in the chapters on morning sickness and motion sickness, but suffice it to say that for nausea and vomiting, ginger is many good herbalists' herb of choice.

Powdered ginger makes a pleasant-tasting tea, but when you're experiencing nausea, nothing seems to do the trick quite as well as ginger ale. Just check the label to make sure that it is made with real ginger; many ginger ales are artificially flavored.

★ **Silence queasiness with cinnamon.** My wife takes cinnamon tea when she feels nauseated. It helps, and I'm not surprised. Cinnamon contains chemicals called catechins, which help relieve nausea.

Catechins also occur in agrimony, barley, bilberries, chinaberries, dog rose, English oak, hops, hawthorn, motherwort, northern red oak, olives, pears, pecans, sage, strawberries, tea and white willow.

★ **Stop spasms with peppermint.** Peppermint tea is a powerful antispasmodic, meaning that it stops muscle spasms in the digestive tract, including those involved in vomiting. (But I wouldn't drink much of it if you're pregnant, since some herbalists have noted that large amounts of peppermint tea may lead to miscarriage.)

Osteoporosis

Osteoporosis, as you probably know, is a disease caused by loss of the mineral calcium and involves a weakening of bone. It is one of the most common conditions associated with aging, and it affects many more women than men.

Osteoporosis causes a variety of possible symptoms: lower back pain, loss of height (up to several inches), stooped posture (dowager's hump) and increased risk of fractures, particularly of the hip.

Until quite recently, the Food and Drug Administration and most physicians told us that supplements, including calcium, were a waste of time and money. Now, very belatedly, they tell us that we're not getting enough calcium. According to the 1995 National Institutes of Health (NIH) Consensus Development Panel on Optimal Calcium Intake, Americans (especially women) should get 1,000 to 1,500 milligrams a day. Unfortunately, most get much less than that, and many don't get even half that amount.

Ironically, the very doctors and federal officials on the NIH panel who would have said "food over supplements" a few years ago now seem to be saying "supplements over food" when it comes to calcium.

The panel did say that, ideally, people should get their calcium from foods such as low-fat dairy products, broccoli, tofu, kale, legumes, canned fish, nuts and seeds. But the panel's report also implied that this is impossible or at least impractical for the vast majority of Americans. The report spent a good deal of space telling people how to take calcium supplements—between meals, to minimize interference with iron absorption.

I have nothing against calcium supplements, but I firmly believe that everyone should get as much calcium as possible from foods.

The other news about osteoporosis that few people know is that high-protein diets leach calcium from bone. Nutrition experts I rely on suggest that people at risk for osteoporosis limit their protein intake to no more than one gram of protein per kilogram of body weight, which translates into around two to three ounces of protein—on the order of one chicken breast—daily for the average woman. Most Americans eat considerably more protein than this, thus running a risk of calcium loss even if they consume a lot of the mineral.

If you're looking to consume less protein and more nutrients that help prevent osteoporosis, here are the plant foods I'd suggest.

★★★ **Use your head—consume cabbage.** Boron helps raise estrogen levels in the blood, and estrogen helps preserve bone. In my database, cabbage ranks highest in boron content among leafy veggies with 145 parts per million (ppm) on a dry-weight basis.

I eat a lot of coleslaw, and it's easy to combine cabbage with high-calcium broccoli, kale, beans and tofu in salads and steamed vegetable dishes.

★★★ **Give this weed a chance.** Speaking of boron, dandelion shoots run a close second to cabbage, with 125 ppm. Dandelion also has more than 20,000 ppm of calcium, meaning that just ten grams (just under seven tablespoons) of dried dandelion shoots could provide more than 1 milligram of boron and 200 milligrams of calcium.

Dandelion is also a fair source of silicon, which some studies suggest also helps strengthen bone.

★★★ **Increase your calcium intake with pigweed.** On a dry-weight basis, pigweed leaves are one of our best vegetable sources of calcium, at 5.3 percent. This means that a small serving of steamed leaves (⅓ ounce or ⅒ cup) provides a hearty 500 milligrams of calcium.

Other good plant sources of calcium, in descending order of potency, include lamb's-quarters, broad beans, watercress, licorice, marjoram, savory, red clover shoots, thyme, Chinese cabbage (bok choy), basil, celery seed, dandelion and purslane.

Overweight

A few years back, a *USA Today* reporter interviewed me about natural secrets of weight control. For the most part, there are no secrets: Just eat a low-fat diet heavy on fruits, vegetables, herbs and whole grains and get plenty of exercise.

You might try these herbs that may help people control their weight.

★★★ **Precede each meal with a psyllium drink.** Plantain is a leafy plant, and psyllium is the seed of the plant. In one Italian study, scientists gave women who were seriously obese—at least 60 percent over their recommended weight—three grams of plantain in water 30 minutes before meals. The plantain group lost more weight than a similar group of women who simply cut back on their diet.

Russian researchers have found that the weight-loss effect of plantain and psyllium is related to the spongy fiber (mucilage) in the seeds and to specific chemicals (polyphenols) in the leaves.

It may not be practical to make a plantain-in-water mixture, but getting psyllium is no problem at all, since Metamucil and similar products contain psyllium. Just mix a teaspoonful with juice or water and have it before each meal. You should watch how you react to this herb if you have allergies, however. If allergic symptoms develop after you take it once, don't use it again.

★★★ **Fight fat with fire.** In one experiment, researchers at Oxford Polytechnic Institute in England measured the metabolic rates of people on a standardized diet, then added a teaspoon of red-pepper sauce and a teaspoon of mustard to every meal. The study showed that the hot herbs raised metabolic rates by as much as 25 percent.

If you're trying to lose weight, you get another benefit from eating spicy foods. The hot spice stimulates thirst, so you drink more liquids. If you fill up on water instead of food, you'll obviously take in fewer calories and gain less weight.

So hot, spicy foods just might help you keep your weight down. One caveat, though: Many people use hot spices in barbecue sauce on high-fat foods such as spareribs, hot dogs and sausages. If you have a yen for barbecue sauce, skip the fat with my Hot Doggone. To a hot dog bun, add coleslaw, barbecue sauce, mustard and onions. I know it sounds weird, but this concoction is surprisingly satisfying. (It's best to leave out the hot dog, but if you must have one, make it vegetarian.)

★★ **Shed pounds with chickweed.** This herb has quite a folk reputation as a slimmer. Try adding some to your diet and see what happens.

Some people eat it raw in salads, and some steam it and eat it like a vegetable. Personally, I prefer to disguise it by including it with other greens. If you want to try my Weed Feed mixture of slimming, edible weeds, mix chickweed, dandelion, evening primrose, stinging nettle (cooked and cooled), plantain and purslane. You can eat this mixture of fresh herbs in a salad. You can also cook all of the greens and perhaps spice them up with slimming hot sauce.

Pain

Doctors recognize two kinds of pain, acute and chronic. Acute pain comes on suddenly, typically subsides with time and usually is alleviated with common pain relievers. Examples would be a headache or the pain of an injury. Chronic pain may begin as acute pain, but it lasts much longer—months or even years—and often cannot be relieved using standard therapies. Those with chronic pain often wind up in a personal hell. Their pain can make them depressed, and with depression the pain may become worse and be more difficult to treat.

If you have persistent pain, see a doctor for a diagnosis. Once the cause has been figured out, rational treatment becomes possible.

There are also a number of herbs that can help.

★★★ **Soothe a toothache with clove oil.** Dentists around the country recommend clove oil as first aid for toothache, and in fact, it's what my mother used to give me for toothache. It works, and its use is endorsed by Commission E, the group that advises the German gonvernment on herbal medicine. You apply this oil directly to the painful tooth.

★★★ **Find relief in red pepper.** Red pepper contains pain-relieving salicylates, chemicals that are similar to salicin, the herbal equivalent of aspirin. In fact, red pepper once ranked as the best food-grade source of salicylates, although a new study has downgraded it considerably. This herb also contains capsaicin, a compound that stimulates the release of the body's natural painkillers, called endorphins.

Some folks like the spicy taste of red pepper. I know I do. I suggest using more of this wonderful spice in your cooking.

Capsaicin also works when used externally by interfering with substance P, a pain transmitter in the skin. So many studies have shown benefits from applying capsaicin externally that the Food and Drug Administration approved pain-relieving skin creams containing 0.025 percent capsaicin (Zostrix, Capzasin-P) for the treatment of arthritis and rheumatism. (If you use a capsaicin cream, be sure to wash your hands thoroughly afterward: You don't want to get it in your eyes. Also, since some people are quite sensitive to this compound, you should test it on a small area of skin to make sure that it's okay for you to use before using it on a larger area. If it seems to irritate your skin, discontinue use.)

★★★ **Whip pain with willow.** Willow bark contains salicin. Just 100 years ago, aspirin was derived from several plants that contain more of these compounds than most: willow, meadowsweet and wintergreen.

Commission E recognizes willow bark as an effective pain reliever for everything from headache to arthritis.

For many kinds of pain relief, I'd start with about a half-teaspoon of salicin-rich willow bark or up to as much as five teaspoons of white willow (*Salix alba*), which has a lower salicin concentration. Of course, not everyone knows which species they have, and salicin content varies from species to species. So I'd suggest starting with a low-dose tea and working your way up to a dose that provides effective pain relief.

If you're allergic to aspirin, you probably shouldn't take aspirin-like herbs, either. Also, you should not give either aspirin or its natural herbal alternatives to children who have pain with viral infections such as colds or flu. There's a chance that they might develop Reye's syndrome, a potentially fatal condition that damages the liver and brain.

Poison Ivy, Poison Oak, and Poison Sumac

Most but not all Americans are sensitive to the irritating oil, urushiol, that's found in plants like poison ivy, poison oak and poison sumac. Those who are sensitive develop a nasty, persistent, blistering rash after contact. It's not clear why some people are relatively or even completely immune to these oils. While it's estimated that some 350,000 Americans experience an episode of poison-plant rash each year, I suspect that figure is low. Many people never call their doctors, so it's hard to get a decent estimate.

The traditional drugstore remedy for reactions to poisonous plants is calamine lotion. It cools the hot rash and relieves some of the itching. But personally, I think several herbal approaches work even better.

★★★ **To prevent a rash, rub on jewelweed.** When poison ivy grows into a sizable clump, I go out and grab a bunch of jewelweed, a succulent, orange-flowered annual that grows in moist meadows on my land. I crush a ball of it in my hands and rub myself down with its juice. Then I spend 15 or 20 minutes pulling up the poison ivy, rubbing myself with jewelweed juice periodically. The result? I never get a poison ivy rash.

★★ **Speed healing with aloe.** The gel inside leathery aloe leaves has been shown again and again to help heal burns and other skin problems. Herbalists also recommend using it to help soothe and heal the rash that follows contact with poisonous plants. If I got a rash that I suspected came from a poisonous plant, I'd slit open a fresh aloe leaf and wipe the gel on the affected area.

★★ **Scratch itching with plantain.** The prestigious *New England Journal of Medicine* reported that poultices made from plantain leaves can help control the itching of poison ivy.

Premenstrual Syndrome

Premenstrual syndrome (PMS) describes a variety of possible symptoms that can occur as a woman approaches menstruation: anxiety, bloating, breast tenderness, irritability, moodiness and weight gain. Most authorities believe that all of these symptoms are caused by changes in the levels of female sex hormones, estrogen and progesterone, that precede menstruation.

The higher the estrogen level, scientists say, the greater the risk of PMS. Estimates vary, but some 25 to 50 percent of menstruating women suffer some degree of PMS, with 8 to 15 percent experiencing severe symptoms.

Fortunately, there are any number of herbs that can help relieve the symptoms.

★★★ **Balance hormones with chasteberry.** The small fruits of the chaste tree have been used for menstrual disorders since Greco-Roman times.

Researchers have found that chasteberry helps relieve PMS because of its effects on female sex hormones. It helps balance hormones produced during women's monthly cycles, increasing production of luteinizing hormone and inhibiting the release of follicle-stimulating hormone. This leads to a shift in the estrogen-progesterone ratio, resulting in less estrogen to cause or aggravate PMS.

The only caveat is that women who have PMS with significant depression should probably steer clear of chasteberry. Some research suggests that PMS with depression is caused by excess progesterone, and chasteberry is said to raise progesterone levels.

For most women, though, chasteberry works. In one year-long study, women with PMS took either 175 milligrams a day of chasteberry extract or 200 milligrams a day of vitamin B_6, a frequently touted supplement that is said to quell PMS. Chasteberry proved clearly superior to the B_6.

At least one chasteberry product is approved in Germany for use as a treatment for PMS, menstrual complaints and breast tenderness. You can buy both the herb itself and herbal tinctures in many stores that carry herbal products.

★★★ **Discourage cramping with Chinese angelica.** One of the most respected herbs in Chinese traditional medicine, Chinese angelica, or *dang gui*, is used primarily as a women's tonic to treat PMS and menstrual cramps. Many women take two capsules twice a day to prevent PMS. (You should not use Chinese angelica if you are pregnant.)

★★★ **Minimize symptoms with evening primrose.** For centuries, American Indian women have been chewing the seeds of the evening primrose for premenstrual and menstrual complaints. And evening primrose is an approved PMS treatment in Great Britain.

I'm not the only herb lover who touts evening primrose for PMS. The word is getting out. On my last pharmacy ecotour to Costa Rica, I overheard a conversation between two women pharmacists who did not know that I was within earshot. One said she took one capsule of evening primrose oil a day all month until she felt her PMS coming on, then upped her intake to four capsules a day until her period was over. She said she'd been doing this for several years and had persuaded all of her co-workers, five other women, to adopt the same regimen.

Prostate Enlargement

The prostate is a small gland that only men have. It sits just above the rectum and provides a good deal of the fluid in semen. Unlike most body parts, the prostate gland grows larger as men age, a condition known as benign prostatic hypertrophy (BPH). By age 40, 10 percent of men have some degree of prostate enlargement. But at age 50, the figure is 50 percent, and it keeps increasing as the years pass. Why is this cause for concern?

The male urethra, the tube through which urine passes, is encircled by the prostate gland. As the prostate grows larger, it pinches the urethra, causing BPH symptoms. It becomes harder to urinate forcefully, and men with BPH have difficulty emptying the bladder completely. The hallmark symptom is having to get up at night to urinate.

I'm betting my own prostate gland that herbal treatments work better than the most commonly prescribed drugs or surgery for controlling BPH, also called noncancerous prostate enlargement. Here are a few of the herbs that I believe provide the best results.

★★★ **Rely on licorice.** Licorice contains a compound that prevents the conversion of testosterone to dihydrotestosterone. Taking very large doses of licorice for a long period of time can produce headache, lethargy, sodium and water retention, excessive loss of potassium and high blood pressure. Some 25 cases have been documented in the world medical literature, and the people who developed problems ate two to four ounces of real licorice candy a day for years.

I doubt that licorice extract would cause any problems. I've personally experienced no symptoms. But if you try the herbal approach to BPH, be alert to any symptoms and cut down drastically on your licorice intake if you experience them.

★★★ **Protect your prostate with pumpkin.** Pumpkin seeds were the traditional treatment for BPH in Bulgaria, Turkey and the Ukraine. The recommendation was a handful of seeds a day throughout adulthood.

The fatty oil in pumpkin seeds is a powerful diuretic, a fact that has caused some nay-sayers to assert that any increased urine flow has nothing to do with relief from BPH. Pumpkin seeds, however, also contain chemicals called cucurbitacins that appear to prevent some transformation of testosterone into dihydrotestosterone.

In addition, pumpkin seeds can contain as much as eight milligrams of zinc per half-cup serving. Naturopaths Joseph Pizzorno, N.D., president of Bastyr University in Seattle, and Michael Murray, N.D, co-authors of *A Textbook of Natural Medicine*, suggest taking 60 milligrams of zinc per day for treating BPH. (This is much more than the Daily Value, so be sure to check with a doctor before you begin taking this much zinc.)

Zinc has been shown to reduce the size of the prostate, presumably by inhibiting the conversion process mentioned earlier. Pumpkin seeds are also high in certain amino acids—alanine, glycine and glutamic acid. Dr. Murray and Dr. Pizzorno report that in a study of 45 men who were given supplements of these amino acids (200 milligrams of each) every day, the regimen significantly relieved BPH symptoms.

A half-cup serving of pumpkin seeds can have 1,150 to 1,245 milligrams of alanine, 1,800 to 1,930 milligrams of glycine and 4,315 to 4,635 milligrams of glutamic acid. That's anywhere from 5 to 20 times the doctors' daily recommendation.

★★★ **Consider saw palmetto.** Shortly after the prescription drug Proscar was approved by the Food and Drug Administration (FDA), the agency banned all nonprescription drugs for BPH. The ban was imposed for two reasons, according to Varro Tyler, Ph.D., dean and professor emeritus of pharmacognosy (natural product pharmacy) at Purdue University in West Lafayette, Indiana. First, the FDA said that no credible evidence was presented to show that any over-the-counter (OTC) products were effective. Second, the agency expressed the view that people who used the OTCs might delay getting proper medical treatment as their condition worsened.

"What the FDA overlooked," says Dr. Tyler, "was the considerable evidence in Western Europe that certain phytomedicinals (plant-based medicines) are effective in treating BPH and that people using them experience an appreciable increase in their comfort level. Perhaps the most popular of these is saw palmetto. . . . The beneficial effects include increased urinary flow, reduced residual urine and decreased frequency of urination."

To date, a half-dozen well-designed studies have shown the effectiveness of saw palmetto. In one study, a clinical trial involving more than 2,000 Germans with BPH, a daily dose of one to two grams of saw palmetto seeds (or 320 milligrams of its hexane extract) produced substantial easing of BPH symptoms.

Raynaud's Disease

Raynaud's disease seems to be caused by constriction and spasms of the small arteries (arterioles) that bring blood to the fingers. As blood flow diminishes, the fingers become painful and turn white or bluish. Raynaud's also occasionally occurs in the nose and toes. It is much more common among women.

While Raynaud's may occur independently of other conditions, sometimes it's a symptom of scleroderma, a rare and serious disease that involves hardening of the skin and damage to the internal organs. Doctors often prescribe corticosteroids such as prednisone (Deltasone, Orasone) to treat both Raynaud's and scleroderma. But corticosteroids have many potentially troubling side effects, such as weight gain, acne and irregular heartbeat. And they sometimes make Raynaud's disease worse.

Because of the problems sometimes caused by corticosteroids, I think it makes a lot more sense to treat Raynaud's with medicinal herbs.

★★★ **Ease the ache with evening primrose.** The oil made from evening primrose contains a good deal of gamma-linolenic acid (GLA). Some studies suggest that GLA helps relieve symptoms of Raynaud's disease.

In one study, evening primrose oil was massaged into the fingers of people with Raynaud's disease. About half improved, more than you would expect if this were simply a placebo response. I suspect that both the massage and the evening primrose oil helped.

★★★ **Enhance circulation with garlic.** Garlic works to improve circulation. In fact, more than one alternative medicine advocate suggests using garlic and ginkgo, which is also known to help circulation, in combination to treat Raynaud's disease. I suggest simply adding more garlic to your diet. You can also take capsules, if you prefer.

★★★ **Make blood flow with ginkgo.** Literally dozens of studies show that ginkgo improves blood circulation. Most of the research has focused on this herb's ability to promote blood flow through the brain, which is why ginkgo extract is widely prescribed in Europe for recovery from stroke and the mental slowing of old age.

But several studies have explored ginkgo's effects on intermittent claudication. When people who have severe claudication take ginkgo, over time the herb improves their ability to walk. While the reasons for the impaired circulation are different, Raynaud's is somewhat similar to claudication, except that it affects the fingers instead of the legs.

European physicians frequently recommend ginkgo for Raynaud's, and there are many European case reports of people with Raynaud's experiencing improvement after taking it. It makes sense to me. If I had this condition, I would try ginkgo.

The medicinal part of the plant is the leaf, but the active constituents (ginkgolides) occur in such low concentration that there's little point in using the leaves to make tea. If you want to try this herb, buy ginkgo pills or capsules made from standardized extract. It's usually a 50:1 ratio, meaning that 50 pounds of ginkgo leaves are processed to yield 1 pound of extract. Look for these extracts in health food stores and herb shops. You can try 60 to 240 milligrams a day, but don't go any higher than that. In large amounts, ginkgo may cause diarrhea, irritability and restlessness.

Sciatica

Sciatica is a condition that involves pain that runs from the lower back to the buttocks and/or the outer back of the leg. It radiates along the sciatic nerve, hence the name. Sometimes the sciatic nerve fibers also become inflamed.

There are a number of herbs that might prove helpful in relieving this kind of pain.

★★★ **Soak in a hayseed bath.** Many years ago, the European naturopath Parson Kneipp learned what people in the Alps did with the seed heads of the various grasses that they stored as hay to feed their animals through the winter. They swept up the hayseed and added it to baths, because they had discovered that this seed has the ability to soothe painful backs, joints and muscles. Kneipp popularized the use of hayseed for this purpose, and today many Europeans subscribe to Kneipp therapy, using hayseed that has been packaged in bath bags or prepared in the form of hot poultices.

But how does hayseed work? It contains a good deal of a compound called coumarin, a camphorlike substance that boosts local blood flow when applied externally, according to Rudolph Fritz Weiss, M.D., Germany's leading herbal physician. (Dr. Weiss's book, *Herbal Medicine*, is used in German medical schools.)

I've heard pretty amazing testimonials endorsing hayseed baths and poultices for relieving sciatic pain. If I had sciatica, I would probably give this approach a try. Ask for Kneipp therapy at specialty bath or herb shops.

★★★ **Stop pain with stinging nettle.** People have been flailing their bad backs with the stinging nettle plant since Roman times. This is a practice that involves taking sprigs of the fresh plant and slapping it against the painful area.

Be warned, though: This practice stings like crazy. But that is part of the treatment. The sting is a counterirritant, something that causes minor pain and in effect fools the nervous system into disregarding deeper pain. That's not all that stinging nettle does, however. Chemicals in the stingers that cause inflammation seem to trigger the release of the body's natural anti-inflammatory chemicals. So the body's own medicine helps get rid of the sciatic inflammation.

Poultices made from stinging nettle are also good for sciatica, according to Dr. Weiss. (Remember that you need to wear gloves whenever you handle this plant to protect your palms from the stingers.)

★★★ **Go wild for willow.** Willow bark contains salicin, the herbal equivalent of aspirin. It can help relieve sciatic pain, and it is recognized as an effective pain reliever for everything from headache to arthritis.

The salicin content of willow varies from species to species. I suggest starting with a low-dose tea made with a half-teaspoon of dried herb and working your way up to a dose that provides effective pain relief.

As with aspirin, long-term use of willow bark may cause stomach distress and even ulcers, so I suggest sweetening willow bark tea with a little licorice, which has ulcer-preventing benefits. And if you're allergic to aspirin, you probably shouldn't take herbal aspirin, either.

Shingles

Shingles is chicken pox returned to haunt you. Like that most common of childhood illnesses, shingles is caused by the herpesvirus. After chicken pox clears up, the virus remains in the body, lying dormant in nerve cells. For reasons that remain a mystery, it can reemerge decades later as shingles.

Symptoms include a painful rash that usually appears on the torso or face. After a few days, chicken pox–like blisters form, then they crust over and eventually heal after two or three weeks. So far it sounds a lot like the childhood disease. In about half of those who develop shingles, however, the pain persists for months and sometimes years. This is called postherpetic neuralgia. Frequently, the pain is quite severe.

Shingles is especially common in people over 60 or those with poor immune function, such as people who are undergoing cancer chemotherapy. If you develop shingles, you should see your doctor immediately for treatment.

Nature has given us several herbs that can help treat viral illnesses. If I developed shingles, I would try any of these approaches.

★★★ **Heal sores with lemon balm.** Herbalists recommend many herbs that are members of the mint family, especially lemon balm, or melissa, to treat herpes. There's good reason for this. Lemon balm has been proven to have some effect on viruses of the herpes family. Varro Tyler, Ph.D., dean and professor emeritus of pharmacognosy (natural product pharmacy) at Purdue University in West Lafayette, Indiana, suggests using lemon balm to treat viral infections.

Herpes cold sores are caused by a virus that behaves much like the virus that causes shingles; in fact, both viruses belong to the same genus. In one well-designed study of 116 people with herpes sores, a lemon balm cream healed the sores substantially better than an inactive cream (a placebo).

For shingles, I'd suggest trying a mixed mint tea made with lots of lemon balm plus any other mints that you have on hand: hyssop, oregano, peppermint, rosemary, sage, self-heal, spearmint or thyme. Put a little licorice in the tea as well. Such a beverage would contain quite a few antiviral, anti-herpetic compounds. I suggest drinking the tea as well as applying it directly to the rash.

★★★ **Rout pain with red pepper.** The fiery ingredient in red pepper, capsaicin, is the hottest thing going for postherpetic neuralgia. Capsaicin brings relief by blocking pain signals from nerves just under the skin. Studies of an ointment containing capsaicin showed such good results that a few years ago, the Food and Drug Administration approved commercial creams such as Zostrix and Capzasin-P, which contain this substance.

You can buy the commercial products if you want. But if you'd like to save money, simply mix powdered red pepper into any white skin lotion until it turns pinkish, then dab it on. Be sure to wash your hands thoroughly afterward so that you don't get pepper in your eyes or on other sensitive areas. And test it on a small area of skin first; if it causes irritation, discontinue use.

Sinusitis

Sinusitis is inflammation, and almost always infection, of the air-filled bony cavities surrounding the nasal passages. It typically develops following a cold or a bout of hay fever. It may also be associated with a dental infection. Mucus fills the sinuses and then becomes infected, typically with bacteria: haemophilus, pneumococcus, staphylococcus or streptococcus.

Sinusitis causes nasal congestion, sometimes severe pain across the nose and cheeks and often a headache as well. Only a small fraction of colds progress to sinusitis. But in susceptible people, almost anything that starts as a cold can turn into a sinus infection.

There are a number of herbs that can help treat this condition.

★★★ **Try nature's infection-fighters—garlic and onion.** These related herbs are broad-spectrum antibiotics. Garlic is the more potent, but onion still rates in my book. Many studies have confirmed garlic's antibiotic activity, most recently a study of people with AIDS who took the herb to ward off all sorts of opportunistic infections, including sinusitis.

Take capsules if you like, but I prefer to peel and chop whole garlic cloves and use them as food. Naturopath Jane Guiltinan, N.D., chief medical officer at Bastyr University in Seattle, feels the same way.

★★★ **Go for the goldenseal.** This is another powerful broad-spectrum herbal antibiotic, with at least two active constituents, berberine and hydrastine. Naturopaths Michael Murray, N.D., and Joseph Pizzorno, N.D., president of Bastyr University, call goldenseal the most effective botanical treatment for acute bacterial infection. I'd have to agree. Lately I've combined goldenseal with echinacea and used it to treat all sorts of minor infections. In fact, I carry it in my travel first-aid kit.

★★ **Enhance immunity with echinacea.** Native to the American Plains, this herb was a favorite American Indian remedy for all sorts of infections. German researchers have shown beyond any doubt that echinacea is an immune stimulant that speeds the healing of bacterial, fungal and viral infections. Studies in other countries support these findings.

Skin Problems

Every winter, the baseboard hot-water radiators in our home make the air very dry. And every year, I develop a skin irritation that I call dry winter dermatitis. Over the years, I've found a skin lotion that helps. Its ingredients are water, glycerin and aloe vera, the traditional and very effective herbal treatment for many skin problems. That's my personal herbal success story.

Herbal approaches have a great deal to offer those with skin problems. In some cases, the herbs help even when pharmaceuticals do not. Here are several of the most helpful herbs.

★★★ **Apply generous amounts of aloe.** Aloe has been used since the days of Egypt's ancient pharaohs to treat all manner of skin problems. But aloe is more than an age-old folk remedy. Since the 1930s, when the gel inside aloe's leathery leaves was shown to speed the healing of radiation burns, many studies have shown this herb to be effective in treating a variety of skin problems. In one study of people undergoing dermabrasion, a medical procedure involving removal of the top layer of skin, aloe speeded healing by 72 hours.

Even if you have a brown thumb, aloe is easy to maintain as a potted plant. It requires little water and almost no care. For minor burns, cuts and other skin problems, simply snip off a lower leaf, slit it open lengthwise, scoop out the gelatinous pulp and apply it to the affected area. Or try one of the many commercial skin products that contain this herb.

★★★ **Ease irritation with evening primrose.** Evening primrose oil is rich in a compound called gamma-linolenic acid (GLA), which is approved in Great Britain for treating eczema. Research I've reviewed supports this use and suggests that this herbal oil is also helpful in treating other forms of skin irritation (dermatitis).

Although evening primrose is a weed at my place, I buy evening primrose oil in capsules at a health food store, and I suggest that this is the easiest way to take this herb. Take the capsules orally, following the package directions. You can also take oils of borage, currant and hops, which are also well-endowed with GLA. As with evening primrose, you can get these other oils in capsule form; follow the package directions when you take them.

★★ **Soothe skin with avocado oil.** There's more to avocado than guacamole. Its oil is actually patented as a treatment for some forms of dermatitis and arthritis. According to Aubrey Hampton, author of *Natural Organic Hair and Skin Care*, long-term treatment with avocado oil helps relieve eczema. I'm not surprised, as avocado oil is rich in vitamins A, D and E, all of which help maintain healthy skin. I suggest applying it directly to any itchy, red or irritated areas. It might also be helpful to ingest the oil and use it in salad dressings.

Smoking

Smoking is estimated to cause one-third of all cancer deaths and one-fourth of the fatal heart attacks in the United States. The American Lung Association estimates that 350,000 Americans die every year from smoking. (My own estimate is 500,000.) Forty percent of smokers die before they reach retirement age.

Smoking damages the blood vessels that supply the penis, so men who smoke have an increased risk of impotence. Smoking also damages the capillaries in women's faces, which is why women smokers develop wrinkles years before nonsmokers. (Smoking develops early wrinkles in men's faces, too, but somehow this particular anti-smoking argument seems to score more points with women than with men.)

Years ago, when I kicked the cigarette habit, I didn't know much about herbal medicine. If I were quitting today, I'd use some herbs to help.

★★★ **Use licorice as a cigarette substitute.** I don't have much science here, just a gut belief to back licorice as an anti-smoking aid. I've also heard a lot of positive stories about people kicking the habit with the help of licorice.

How does this work? Licorice root happens to look just like an old cheroot cigar. You can keep a stick of licorice root handy and suck on it in place of a cigarette. I believe it works by helping to satisfy the oral cravings that people who are addicted to cigarettes seem to have. If I were still a smoker, I'd give this one a try.

You should be aware that while licorice and its extracts are safe for normal use in moderate amounts—up to about three cups of tea a day—long-term use (more than six weeks) or ingestion of excessive amounts can produce headache, lethargy, sodium and water retention, excessive loss of potassium and high blood pressure.

★★★ **To control cravings, chew on red clover.** Red clover has an age-old reputation as a cancer preventer. For tumors to grow, they need a blood supply, and they send out biochemical signals that coax the body into growing blood vessels right into them, a process called angiogenesis.

Several leading cancer researchers have been working on ways to stop these new blood vessels from forming, thereby starving tumors. It turns out that one compound with an anti-angiogenic effect is genistein, a constituent of red clover.

Aspiring ex-smokers can chew on fresh clover flowers (you can add them to salads) or anything else that contains genistein, such as groundnuts, peanuts or soybeans. These munchies would help satisfy some of the oral needs that smokers and ex-smokers seem to have. At the same time, the genistein in these snacks would be attacking any tumors that might be trying to get a start.

If you're having a hard time kicking the smoking habit, you might want to develop another habit—drinking red clover tea daily. It seems as if it would offer a measure of protection.

★★ **Combat cancer with carrots.** Back when I quit smoking, carrots helped me quite a bit. I used to drive to the office munching on a raw carrot or two instead of puffing on a cigarette.

At the time, I chose carrots because I like them, but now we know that carotenoids, the chemical relatives of vitamin A that give carrots their orange color, also help prevent cancer, especially if the carotenoids come from carrots or other whole foods rather than from capsules. (Generally, if you isolate one beneficial chemical—take it out of context—you're missing out on a whole lot of other chemistry that can also help.)

If cigarettes are cancer sticks, carrots are *anti*-cancer sticks. In fact, all fruits and vegetables are. The research is consistent and compelling: The more fruits and vegetables people eat, the less likely they are to develop every major cancer, including lung cancer. So even if you don't quit smoking, you should still be munching on carrots.

Sore Throat

Sore throat is a typical first symptom of colds. (Many of the herbal suggestions in the chapter on colds and flu on page 42 apply here as well.) But sore throat may also be caused by exposure to chemical irritants or by streptococcus bacteria (strep throat). If you develop a sore throat with a fever and no other symptoms, it might be strep, and a visit to the doctor is strongly advised.

Most commercial sore throat treatments involve sucking on anesthetic lozenges that deaden the nerve cells in the throat so that you don't feel the pain. I prefer the herbal alternatives, which actually soothe inflamed tissue. Here are the herbs that can help.

★★★ **Shrink swollen tissues with eucalyptus.** Commission E, the body of experts that advises the German government about herbs, approves using eucalyptus to treat sore throat.

Eucalyptus helps in two ways. The aromatic oil has a cooling effect on inflamed tissue, and the tannins in eucalyptus exert soothing astringent action as well. I suggest using a few teaspoons of crushed leaf per cup of boiling water to make a soothing tea.

★★★ **Support healing with honeysuckle.** The Chinese use honeysuckle flowers extensively to treat sore throat, colds, flu, tonsillitis, bronchitis and pneumonia. In one study of 425 Chinese students with strep throats, positive results were obtained with a treatment that involved blowing powdered dried honeysuckle flowers, blackberry lily roots and a small amount of borneol into the backs of their throats. (Borneol is just one of more than 20 antiseptic compounds found in honeysuckle flowers.)

I don't think that you need to use powdered honeysuckle to get the benefit of this herb. Honeysuckle flower extracts are strongly active against many microorganisms that cause sore throat and respiratory conditions.

I personally like using honeysuckle in combination with forsythia flowers for my own sore throats, and I often take them in hot lemonade sweetened with licorice, especially in winter.

★★★ **Relieve irritation with licorice.** Licorice has been revered as a sore throat treatment for centuries in both Europe and China.

Commission E approves licorice for treating sore throat, and its effectiveness has been scientifically documented, according to pharmacognosist (natural product pharmacist) Albert Leung, Ph.D.

Dr. Leung recommends starting with three cups of water and five to seven teaspoons of root pieces. Put the herb in the water and bring it to a boil, then simmer until about half of the water has boiled away.

Licorice not only soothes a sore throat, it also has an expectorant effect that can help treat colds and other respiratory conditions. (Like most non-nutritive sweeteners, licorice has an "off" taste that some people find less than appealing.)

★★★ **Slip away from soreness.** Slippery elm is an all-around soother, helping the throat, the respiratory tract and the digestive tract. And like most if not all woody plants, slippery elm contains compounds called oligomeric procyanidins, which have antiseptic and anti-allergic action.

Sties

A sty is a bacterial infection (typically staphylococcal) of an eyelash follicle. The infection causes a pus-filled bump to form on either the inside or outside of the eyelid. The bump grows for a week or so and then usually subsides, possibly rupturing spontaneously as it heals.

Sties should not be squeezed like pimples, as squeezing can spread the infection. Some people never get sties. Among those who do, they tend to recur.

Doctors often recommend holding a warm, moist cloth against the affected eye to hasten drainage. They also frequently prescribe antibiotics that attack the bacteria.

Herbalists also have two approaches to treatment—antibiotic herbs plus herbs that boost the immune system so that the body can fight the infection more effectively.

★★★ **Battle bacteria with echinacea.** This is one of my favorite immune stimulants. It was widely used to treat infections back in the days before antibiotics, and no wonder: Research clearly demonstrates its immunostimulant properties.

But in addition, this herb of our Great Plains, which is also known as coneflower, has antibacterial properties. Just six milligrams of the active constituents (echinacosides) in echinacea is the antibiotic equivalent of one unit of penicillin, according to herbal pharmacologist Daniel Mowrey, Ph.D., author of *The Scientific Validation of Herbal Medicine* and *Herbal Tonic Therapies*. (A standard dose of penicillin is around 180 units.)

You take this herb orally, either in a tea or in capsules, rather than using it in a compress. (Although echinacea can cause your tongue to tingle or go numb temporarily, this effect is harmless.)

★★★ **Prepare a goldenseal compress.** Like echinacea, goldenseal is both an immune booster and an antibiotic. In one study, berberine, an active constituent in this herb, was shown to be more active against staph infections, the kind that cause sties, than chloramphenicol (Chloromycetin), a powerful pharmaceutical antibiotic.

And berberine is only one of the medicinal compounds in goldenseal and its herb-medicinal relatives, barberry, goldthread, Oregon grape and yellowroot. You can take goldenseal orally, in either tea or capsules, but it also can be helpful when used in a compress.

★★★ **Stymie a sty with potato.** I always like to quote herb conservative Varro Tyler, Ph.D., dean and professor emeritus of pharmacognosy (natural product pharmacy) at Purdue University in West Lafayette, Indiana: "To treat a sty, take fresh scrapings from the inside of a potato, put them on a piece of clean cloth and place on the sty. Replace once or twice with fresh scrapings. . . . It was amazingly effective. Within a couple of hours, the swelling was down, and the sty was significantly improved. By that evening it was almost gone."

If it's good enough for Dr. Tyler, it's good enough for me.

Sunburn

As burns go, most sunburns are comparatively mild. But sunburns cover a lot more of the body than most other everyday burns. And in addition to increasing cancer risk, they can be quite painful. Fortunately, Nature has provided us with several good remedies.

★★★ **Temper the burn with tea.** The Chinese recommend applying cooled black tea to the skin to soothe sunburn. That sounds good to me because of several beneficial chemical compounds that tea contains.

One researcher I know says that the tannic acid and theobromine in tea help remove heat from sunburn. Other compounds in tea called catechins help prevent and repair skin damage and may even help prevent chemical- and radiation-induced skin cancers. The latest studies show that green tea is also high in chemicals called polyphenols. When ingested, these chemicals help protect the skin against damage from the ultraviolet radiation that causes sunburn.

There's no doubt that it's better to avoid sunburn than endure the after-effects. But if you do spend too much time in the sun with not enough sunscreen, soothe the burn by sipping iced green tea. Then apply cool compresses of the tea to any areas of skin that have been overexposed.

★★ **Slather on aloe gel.** The inner gel of the aloe vera leaf has been shown to speed the healing of radiation-induced burns. You can scoop the gel directly from split leaves or buy commercially prepared gel at a health food store or herb shop.

Apply aloe gel after showering, then reapply it a few more times each day until the pain has subsided, suggests cardiac surgeon and sports medicine specialist Robert D. Willix, M.D., of Boca Raton, Florida. Usually, he says, the redness disappears in a day or two, and the skin does not peel.

★★ **Make your own black nightshade cream.** Some Indiana folk herbalists crush nightshade leaves, stir them into heavy cream and pat the mixture on sunburn, notes Varro Tyler, Ph.D., dean and professor emeritus of pharmacognosy (natural product pharmacy) at Purdue University in West Lafayette, Indiana.

I've witnessed a similar practice in the Amazon. A Peruvian shamanistic healer I know uses an Amazonian species of nightshade to treat all manner of burns, not just sunburn. He chops the leaves to express a greenish juice, which he applies to a burn as soon as possible, swearing that it prevents scarring.

If you have access to a black nightshade plant, you might want to give this one a try. Compounds in other species of *Solanum* have proved useful in helping to prevent skin cancer.

Tinnitus

Tinnitus is chronic ringing in the ears, although sometimes the sound is more like a roaring or whooshing. Doctors don't really know what causes tinnitus and often have very little success in alleviating it.

If tinnitus bothers you, don't take aspirin or aspirin-like herbs—willow bark, meadowsweet and wintergreen. High doses of aspirin may cause ringing in the ears. I've also seen reports that a few other herbs may aggravate tinnitus, among them cinchona, black haw and uva ursi.

Fortunately, other natural approaches can help.

★★★ **First, try a ginkgo extract.** Hundreds of European studies have confirmed the use of standardized ginkgo extract for a wide variety of conditions associated with aging, including tinnitus, vertigo, memory loss and poor circulation. Ginkgo does not work in every case of tinnitus, but it is the herb I'd try first.

The active constituents in ginkgo leaf, ginkgolides, occur in concentrations too dilute to allow the use of teas or tinctures. The way to take ginkgo is as a 50:1 standardized extract, meaning that 50 pounds of ginkgo leaves are processed into 1 pound of extract. You'll have to buy this extract in a pharmacy or health food store; look for 50:1 on the label. Most experts recommend taking 40 milligrams of ginkgo extract three times a day to treat tinnitus.

★★ **Nibble on sesame seeds.** Chinese herbalists recommend sesame seeds for the treatment of tinnitus, blurred vision and dizziness. If you'd like to give sesame seeds a try, there's probably no harm in adding it to foods. Or try tahini, the peanut-butter-like spread made from sesame seeds, or halvah, which is sesame candy.

★ **Banish ringing with black cohosh.** In her interesting feminist herbal, *The Roots of Healing*, Deb Soule, distinguished Maine herbalist and founder of Avena Botanicals, spins the tale of a professional flutist neighbor of hers who had been troubled for years by tinnitus. This neighbor took black cohosh tincture for a few weeks, and his tinnitus almost disappeared. He became a disciple of herbalism. Deb adds that black cohosh and ginkgo are a good combination.

Tonsillitis

Tonsillitis is an inflammation of the tonsils, the small round lymph glands sitting on the sides of the throat. It occurs most frequently in children under nine. Usually the tonsils become inflamed because they have been exposed to infection-causing microorganisms, frequently streptococcal bacteria or a virus. If you have tonsillitis, you should see a doctor for treatment. It's especially important to treat a strep infection with antibiotics because this kind of infection can lead to a heart-damaging bout of rheumatic fever.

Tonsillitis—and inflammation of the related glands, the adenoids—shows that the body is defending itself from infection. Here are the herbs that can help fight off the infection and soothe the inflammation.

★★★ **Build your body's defenses with echinacea.** Herbs that enhance immunity are useful in almost all infections. Echinacea, also known as coneflower, is a fine one, according to many European studies. Echinacea stimulates phagocytosis, the devouring of bacteria and viruses by certain types of white blood cells. As with so many mouth and throat infections, I'd recommend going with a double whammy by taking echinacea along with goldenseal, another potent antiseptic, antibiotic and immune stimulant.

★★ **Be generous with garlic.** Garlic is useful in treating any kind of throat infection, including tonsillitis. James Balch, M.D., a urologist, and his wife, Phyllis, a certified nutritional consultant, recommend taking two garlic capsules a day for either sore throat or tonsillitis. (They also suggest eating more of garlic's close relative, onions.)

Capsules are a convenient way to take garlic, but not all experts give them top billing. Jane Guiltinan, N.D., chief medical officer at Bastyr University in Seattle, for example, prefers whole garlic cloves to capsules or extracts. I agree.

May I suggest that my Tonsil Soup is also good for treating tonsillitis? To make it, use any favorite recipe for an onion/garlic soup. Then be very generous with any or all of the hot spices that contain vitamin C and other good sorethroat fighters, including chili pepper, ginger, horseradish, mustard seed and pepper.

★★ **Beat bacteria with honeysuckle.** Honeysuckle flowers are used in China to treat tonsillitis, bronchitis, colds, flu and pneumonia. Extracts made from these flowers act strongly against a broad spectrum of bacteria. It's small wonder, since the flowers contain more than a dozen antiseptic compounds.

In one study, researchers looked at 425 Chinese students with strep throat. This is not tonsillitis, admittedly, but it is a related throat infection. In this study, researchers spurred rapid healing by introducing an herbal preparation that included powdered dried honeysuckle flowers into the backs of the students' throats.

I would not hesitate to use honeysuckle, by itself or combined with forsythia, to treat tonsillitis. In fact, I do use the leaves of both plants to treat many midwinter respiratory infections.

Toothache

There's no need to define toothache. I've suffered quite a few over the years, and to this day, I stupidly procrastinate about going to the dentist. It turns out that I'm not alone. An estimated 98 percent of Americans have dental cavities, according to the National Institute of Dental Research. All this adds up to millions of toothaches a year.

Any persistent toothache should be checked by a dentist. But fortunately, you don't have to suffer on your way there, thanks to some good herbs.

★★★ **Numb pain with clove oil.** Germany's Commission E, the body of natural medicine experts that makes herbal recommendations to that country's counterpart of the Food and Drug Administration (FDA), endorses oil of clove as a local anesthetic and antiseptic for toothache. Even a scientific committee reporting to our FDA commented that oil of clove was the only one of 12 ingredients commonly found in toothache preparations that was "safe and effective for temporary use on a tooth with throbbing pain." Oil of clove contains a great deal of the anesthetic, antiseptic chemical eugenol. Cloves are 5 to 20 times richer in eugenol than other eugenol sources listed in my database.

You can buy over-the-counter preparations of clove oil to use yourself to numb toothache. The oil is placed directly on the tooth, not ingested.

★★ **Tame the ache with ginger.** A compress made with this hot spice seems to help alleviate toothache pain. I'd add more heat to such a compress myself, in the form of red pepper. Both ginger and red pepper seem to work like the old mustard plasters. They act as counterirritants, meaning that the surface irritation of the ginger or red pepper helps to diminish the deeper toothache pain.

To make a compress for your tooth, mix the powdered spice or spices in enough water to form a gooey paste. Then dip in a small cotton ball and wring it out. Apply the cotton directly to the tooth without letting it touch your gum. If you can't stand the heat, rinse your mouth and try some other remedy.

★★ **Feel better with red pepper.** In 1992, while the world celebrated Columbus's voyage, I celebrated the introduction of red pepper outside America. Columbus was introduced to the spice by the Caribbean Indians.

When applied to the skin, capsaicin, the hot ingredient in red pepper, burns for a while, but it depletes the action of substance P, the chemical in the body responsible for transmitting pain. In addition, red pepper is fairly well endowed with salicylates, aspirin-like chemicals that can relieve pain. It's no wonder that this herb is an old folk remedy for toothache. To use red pepper on a toothache, use the cotton compress technique described for ginger.

Tooth Decay

An estimated 98 percent of Americans have cavities; most develop between the ages of 5 and 15. Researchers believe that cavity formation drops off by the midteens because the body develops immunity to decay-causing bacteria, primarily several types of streptococcus.

Tooth decay was an even bigger problem before the fluoridation of water in this century. From ancient times until the nineteenth century, herbalists put a great deal of effort into studying plants that helped preserve teeth. They discovered quite a few that were very effective.

★★★ **Discourage decay with tea.** In addition to a generous endowment of several compounds that work together to prevent tooth decay, tea also contains a considerable amount of tooth-preserving fluoride.

Green tea may contain more fluoride than black tea. To get potent decay-preventive action from just the fluoride in tea, you'd have to drink three to ten cups a day. But you actually need less because of all the other anti-cavity compounds in tea. (There's also a good chance that the water you use for your tea already contains fluoride.) If you sweeten your tea, try using licorice instead of decay-promoting sugar. To do this, simply brew your regular tea with a little dried licorice root.

★★ **Destroy bacteria with bay.** Bay's aromatic oil contains a powerful bacteria-killing chemical (1,8-cineole) that is used in some dentifrices. Check the toothpaste label for bay if you'd like to take advantage of this herb's decay-preventing potential. If you don't find a toothpaste containing this ingredient in your pharmacy, you might have better luck at your local health food store.

★★ **Look for toothpaste made with bloodroot.** Many studies have shown that dental-care products containing bloodroot help reduce the amount of dental plaque deposited on the teeth in as little as eight days. Bloodroot contains a compound known as sanguinarine, which seems to be responsible for the plaque-reducing effect.

Sanguinarine chemically binds to dental plaque and helps prevent it from adhering to the teeth. And since dental plaque is responsible for gum disease as well as tooth decay, bloodroot is also a good choice for adults who are fighting gum disease.

You can take advantage of bloodroot's plaque-fighting potential by looking for toothpastes and mouthwashes that contain this herb. One popular brand is Viadent.

Ulcers

Technically, an ulcer is any sore. But when people say that they have an ulcer, they almost always mean an internal sore in the lining of the stomach or duodenum, the gateway to the small intestine just downstream from the stomach.

These kinds of ulcers are also called peptic ulcers because they occur in areas that are exposed to the digestive enzyme pepsin.

An estimated 10 percent of Americans have an ulcer at some point in life, with about one million new diagnoses a year. Men are four times more susceptible than women, and risk rises with age. Allergies somehow make people more ulcer-prone: In one study, 98 percent of people with peptic ulcers also had respiratory allergies.

Not long ago, scientists thought that stress caused ulcers. It may well play a role, but now we know that the real culprit is often an infection caused by the bacteria *Helicobacter pylori*, sometimes known as *Campylobacter pylori*. Simply having *H. pylori* bacteria in your system doesn't mean that you will get an ulcer. However, more than 75 percent of people with ulcers show evidence of *H. pylori* infection, and that's straight from the pages of the *Journal of the American Medical Association*.

These days, doctors generally treat ulcers caused by *H. pylori* with a combination of antibiotics plus bismuth (Pepto-Bismol) or similar drugs. In addition, you might try a number of herbal anti-ulcer approaches.

★★★ **Hit ulcers with a ginger-honey combination.** How about candied ginger as an herbal alternative to cimetidine (Tagamet), ranitidine (Zantac) and famotidine (Pepcid)? It would sure taste a lot better!

Ginger is well-known for its anti-inflammatory activity, but it's considerably less known as an herbal treatment for ulcers. In fact, ginger contains 11 compounds that have demonstrated anti-ulcer effects.

Eating honey-candied ginger is a pleasant-tasting treatment for ulcers, according to Paul Schulick, New England herbalist and author of *Ginger: Common Spice and Wonder Drug*. The combination of honey and ginger is particularly effective, he notes. In addition to the antibacterial compounds that are available from ginger, honey has antibacterial action, and the two together seem to produce synergistic effects.

★★★ **Speed healing with licorice.** German physicians have always been more open to herbal medicine than doctors in the United States, and they have researched herbal alternatives extensively. Commission E, the body of scientists that advises the German counterpart of the Food and Drug Administration, approves licorice as an ulcer treatment. This recommendation is based on the medical traditions of Asia, the Middle East and Europe, plus literally dozens of scientific studies.

Licorice contains several anti-ulcer compounds, including glycyrrhizic acid. Licorice and its extracts are safe for normal use in moderate amounts, up to about three cups of tea a day. However, long-term use—daily use for longer than six weeks—or ingestion of excessive amounts can produce symptoms such as headache, lethargy, sodium and water retention, excessive loss of potassium and high blood pressure.

These side effects, however, can be largely eliminated by using a slightly processed form of the herb called deglycyrrhizinated licorice (DGL). In one good study, DGL was at least as effective in speeding ulcer healing as the newest class of pharmaceutical drugs, called histamine-blocking agents, that were designed to do this. DGL also seems to protect the digestive lining from aspirin's ulcer-promoting effects.

Commercial licorice preparations containing DGL are readily available in natural food stores that sell herbs. If you have an ulcer, this is the preferred form of licorice to take, but clearly some of the power of the herb is lost with the lost glycyrrhizin.

If you'd like to take licorice from time to time as an ulcer preventive, you can do what I do. When you're brewing some other herbal tea, add a little licorice. Licorice by itself makes a sweet, pleasant-tasting tea, and when added to other teas, it serves as a sweetener.

★★★ **Get rid of *H. pylori* with yellowroot.** Yellowroot is an antibiotic that should work by helping to control *H. pylori* bacteria. I personally would try a teaspoon of yellowroot tincture in juice or tea once or twice a day before moving on to the antibiotics my doctor might prescribe for ulcer. If you're already taking antibiotics, however, do not make this switch without first discussing it with your doctor.

Varicose Veins

Varicose veins occur when the valves in the veins that prevent blood from flowing backward don't work properly. Blood forms pools, and where this occurs, the veins and nearby capillaries become distended and swollen, leaking blood and fluid into surrounding tissue. This condition occurs most frequently in the legs; in areas where veins are near the surface, it causes unsightly bluish streaks, trails or spidery markings. But this condition can develop elsewhere as well. When they occur in and around the anus, these problem veins (varicosities) are known as hemorrhoids. When they occur in the scrotum, they are known as varicoceles.

Varicose veins affect about 15 percent of Americans, especially women, and the tendency to have this condition seems to run in families. When they occur in the legs, varicose veins are most common on the calves and along the inner thighs.

A number of herbs can help prevent or treat this problem.

★★★ **Strengthen veins with horse chestnut.** In traditional herbal medicine, horse chestnut seeds were used to treat varicose veins and hemorrhoids. Eventually, botanists isolated the most active compound, aescin, and experiments with laboratory animals supported its traditional use as a remedy. Aescin helps strengthen capillary cells and reduce fluid leakage.

Commission E, the committee of scientific experts that advises the German counterpart of the Food and Drug Administration, endorses horse chestnut for treating varicose veins. On this side of the Atlantic, Varro Tyler, Ph.D., dean and professor emeritus of pharmacognosy (natural product pharmacy) at Purdue University in West Lafayette, Indiana, is also an advocate. In his excellent book for clinicians, *Herbs of Choice*, he singles out horse chestnut seed as by far the most effective plant drug for treating varicose veins.

In Europe, horse chestnut preparations are marketed as extracts of the leaves, bark and/or seeds, which are taken orally. Like most European plant medicines, horse chestnut extracts are standardized, and the dosage should be on the label. Unfortunately, these standardized extracts are not yet widely available in the United States.

You must obtain a standardized extract and follow package directions if you're going to use horse chestnut as a healing herb. It's simply not safe to use otherwise. If you can't find the extract, you'll have to rely on other herbs mentioned in this chapter.

★★★ **Reinforce vein walls with violet.** Violet flowers contain generous amounts of a compound called rutin, which helps maintain the strength and integrity of capillary walls. Medical texts say that taking 20 to 100 milligrams of rutin daily can significantly strengthen the capillaries.

Are violets safe to eat? Yes. I've eaten 100 or so violet flowers on several different occasions, and I've never suffered any ill effects. Both violets and pansies, which also contain significant amounts of rutin, are usually cited in the books about edible flowers. As far as I can determine, they are safe when consumed at these low levels, and both flowers make impressive additions to salads.

★★★ **Outwit weak veins with witch hazel.** Witch hazel comes in two commercial preparations, water extracts (witch hazel water) and alcohol extracts (tincture of witch hazel). Both are soothingly astringent, which makes witch hazel a popular external herbal treatment for various skin conditions from bruises to varicose veins.

Studies with laboratory animals have shown that this herb helps strengthen blood vessels. Commission E endorses using witch hazel extracts externally to treat both hemorrhoids and varicose veins. Simply wipe the affected area with a cotton ball that has been dipped in the extract.

Tincture of witch hazel can be taken internally for varicose veins, says the *Lawrence Review of Natural Products*, a respected newsletter. Or to make a tea, steep one to two teaspoons of dried witch hazel leaves in a cup of boiling water for ten minutes. You can drink two to three cups a day.

★★ **Sweep away the problem with butcher's broom.** This herb has a long history of treating venous problems like hemorrhoids and varicose veins. It contains two anti-inflammatory compounds, ruscogenin and neoruscogenin, that constrict and strengthen veins.

Viral Infections

Viruses are very strange. They are incredibly small—so tiny that while ordinary microscopes can see the body's cells and the bacteria that may infect them, you need much more powerful electron microscopes to see virus particles.

I use the word *particle* because by most definitions of life, viruses aren't really alive. They contain only genetic material (DNA or RNA) surrounded by a protein capsule. Viruses don't ingest food, breathe oxygen or eliminate wastes. All they do is reproduce after they've infected cells that are susceptible to them.

Antibiotics are generally useless against viruses; they work most actively against bacteria. Since the discovery of penicillin in 1928, mainstream medicine has come up with dozens of antibiotics. But today we still have only a handful of antiviral drugs, among them acyclovir for herpes, AZT for AIDS and interferon, the body's own virus fighter.

The good news is that several herbs used in traditional herbal medicine have scientifically documented antiviral effects. They're what I use when I have colds, flu and other viral infections. I discuss many of these herbs in the chapter on colds and flu (see page 42), but I want to devote one chapter to a look at herbs that can be tried as a treatment for any viral infection.

★★★ **Defeat viruses with echinacea.** This is by far the most popular antiviral herb, and for good reason. Echinacea fights viruses in two ways. It contains three compounds with specific antiviral activity—caffeic acid, chicoric acid and echinacin. Root extracts of echinacea have also been shown to act like interferon, the body's own antiviral compound. In addition, echinacea is an immune stimulant that helps the body defend itself against viral infection more effectively.

Commission E, the German expert committee that judges the value of herbal medicines for the German government, has approved echinacea for treatment of influenza–like symptoms. That constitutes a significant scientific endorsement of this herb, which is native to America.

★★ **Improve immunity with astragalus.** Also known as *huang qi*, this is an immune-boosting herb from China. In one small Chinese study, ten people whose heart muscles were infected by *Coxsackie B* virus, which causes the heart inflammation known as myocarditis, received injections of astragalus extract for three to four months. The activity of their natural killer cells, a component of the immune system, rose 11 to 45 percent. They also showed increased levels of alpha- and gamma-interferon, the body's own antiviral compounds. Not surprisingly, their symptoms improved. European studies suggest that, as with echinacea, many of the immune-stimulating compounds in astragalus are active when taken orally.

★★ **Jump on the juniper bandwagon.** Even among herbalists, it's not widely known that juniper contains a potent antiviral compound (deoxypodophyllotoxin). Juniper extracts appear to inhibit a number of different viruses, including those that cause flu and herpes. Sometimes when I feel a cold coming on, I make a juniper tea.

★★ **Drink a natural antiviral—lemon balm.** Also known as melissa, this herb is highly recommended as an antiviral, especially against herpes. I would try lemon balm for treating any viral infection. It makes a very pleasant tea.

Warts

The common wart is very common indeed. But sometimes it seems as if folk treatments for warts are even more common. There's good reason for this: Not only do many folk treatments work, they often make physicians' treatments look clumsy by comparison.

Warts are benign skin tumors that are caused by at least 35 different members of one family of viruses called papillomavirus. The common wart typically appears on the hand, especially in older children, but warts can occur on other parts of the body as well. (Plantar warts are the kind that show up only on the feet.) Researchers have observed that individuals with suppressed immune systems are far more susceptible to warts than those with normal immunity.

Here are the herbs you might want to consider if you're fighting this annoyingly persistent problem. Some of the substances recommended in this chapter can be quite irritating to the skin. Everyone's skin is different, so if you try one of these remedies and it seems to make the skin around the wart red and irritated, rinse the area thoroughly and discontinue use of the herb.

★★★ **Shrink the bump with birch bark.** Birch bark has been used to treat warts in places as diverse as China, Scandinavia and Michigan. It contains two compounds, betulin and betulinic acid, that have antiviral activity. Birch bark also contains salicylates, which are approved by the Food and Drug Administration (FDA) for treatment of warts.

If you have access to fresh birch bark, you can tape a piece of moistened bark directly to the wart. You can also brew up some birch bark tea by adding a teaspoon or two of powdered bark to a cup of boiling water and steeping for ten minutes. You can drink the tea and also rub it directly on the warts.

★★ **Deliver an herbal one-two punch.** Many people in many countries recommend castor bean oil for warts. They say you should massage the oil directly into the wart several times a day.

There are a number of ways that you might try to give the oil's anti-wart effects a little boost. I'd suggest putting a handful of willow bark into the oil and letting it steep for a couple of days. Willow contains aspirin-like compounds known as salicylates, which might prove helpful. Other herbalists drop in a few cloves of garlic, another folk remedy for warts, and allow the mixture to steep for a few days.

★★ **Kill the virus with celandine.** Celandine contains some of the same compounds as bloodroot (chelerythrine, sanguinarine and proteolytic enzymes). Celandine juice can inhibit the wart virus or even kill it, according to Rudolph Fritz Weiss, M.D., dean of German medical herbalists and author of *Herbal Medicine*. If you have access to the fresh plant, you might apply the yellow juice directly to the wart once or twice a day for five to seven days. Otherwise, you can try applying a strong tea made from the dried herb.

Wrinkles

Wrinkles result from changes in collagen, the protein that makes up the fibrous portion of your skin. Collagen is what holds you together. It makes up about one-third of your body's total protein and 70 percent of your connective tissue.

Young skin and connective tissue contain mostly elastic or soluble collagen, and as a result, it can absorb moisture and plump up. This ongoing process of moisturization and swelling keeps young, elastic skin looking sleek and smooth. But with sun exposure, cigarette smoking and normal aging comes oxidative damage to the skin. This damage is the same sort of thing that happens to iron when it rusts. In the body, this chemical process causes the formation of insoluble collagen, which is inelastic, is unable to absorb water well and does not plump up.

With loss of elasticity and moisture, lines and wrinkles form, especially in areas exposed to sunlight—the face, the neck and the backs of the hands.

Most natural anti-wrinkle treatments rely on antioxidants and emollients. Antioxidants are substances that mop up free radicals, the highly reactive oxygen molecules that are responsible for oxidative damage. Emollients help prevent dryness while moisturizing and softening the skin. Here are some natural treatments that might prove helpful.

★★★ **Fend off free radicals with horse chestnut and witch hazel.** Japanese scientists tested 65 plant extracts and found seven that showed sufficient antioxidant activity to have potential against wrinkles. The four that you probably can get your hands on are horse chestnut, witch hazel, rosemary and sage, but the researchers singled out horse chestnut and witch hazel as the best. Both of these are strong antioxidants. Soothing and astringent salves containing these herbs are available at health food stores, but I prefer to mix them myself.

★★ **For healthy skin, eat carrots.** Carrots are high in vitamin A, and deficiencies of this vitamin cause dry skin and wrinkling. Carrots also contain the antioxidant beta-carotene. I'd suggest munching a carrot or two a day, not only to prevent wrinkles but for all the cancer-preventive chemicals that this vegetable contains.

You might also consider topical application of carrot oil. Its high levels of vitamin A make it a good sunscreen, according to Aubrey Hampton, author of *Natural Organic Hair and Skin Care.* I confess I've never tried carrot oil, but on occasion, I've mashed carrots in a blender and experimentally applied the mash as a face mask. Someone once even called me a handsome old redneck. (Wash the mashed carrot off after 15 to 30 minutes.)

★★ **Look for skin products with cocoa butter.** A major emollient used in skin lotions and cosmetics, cocoa butter is the leading anti-wrinkle suggestion of pharmacognosist (natural product pharmacist) Albert Leung, Ph.D. It melts at body temperature and remoisturizes dry skin, especially around the eyes (crow's-feet), the corners of the mouth and on the neck (turkey neck). I like it because it comes from the Amazon. Another similar tropical emollient is coconut oil.

Yeast Infections

Most people think of yeast infections, also known as candidiasis, as a plague only upon women. But men can also develop candidiasis, especially those who are uncircumcised. A man with yeast typically shows no symptoms, but each time his partner is treated and gets rid of her infection, he reinfects her. So if you're a woman who's been having problems with yeast infections, be sure your partner is checked, too: Both of you might need some of these herbal remedies.

Yeast infection is caused by a group of yeastlike fungi called candida. *Candida albicans* is the most common culprit, but it's not the only one. Everyone has a certain amount of candida living on them and in them, but not everyone develops candidiasis.

Yeast live on moist areas of the body, such as the lining of the mouth and the vagina. They usually cause no problem, but sometimes they overgrow, causing infection. The vagina is the primary site. But yeast infections can also develop in the mouth (thrush), in the respiratory tract (bronchocandidiasis) and on the skin (dermatocandidiasis).

Yeast has become more of problem than it was, say, 60 years ago, because several modern drugs spur yeast overgrowth. Among the leading culprits are antibiotics, steroids and birth control pills.

There are a number of herbs that can help fight yeast infections, but you'd better be sure of what you're dealing with before you self-medicate. If you have what you suspect is a yeast infection, please see your doctor for a diagnosis. Then, if you'd like to try an herbal alternative as your treatment of choice, you should discuss it with her. You might consider using these herbs in addition to whatever is prescribed for you.

★★★ **Defeat infection with echinacea.** This herb's immune-stimulating action seems to be particularly helpful for treating yeast infections. In studies using laboratory animals, treatment with the herb protected mice from *C. albicans* infections. It works by stimulating the white blood cells to gobble up yeast organisms, a process known as phagocytosis.

In an impressive German study, women with recurrent vaginal yeast infections were given either standard antifungal medication or the antifungal plus an echinacea extract. Among those taking just the antifungal, 60 percent suffered recurrences. But among the women taking the drug plus echinacea, only about 10 percent experienced recurrences. That sounds to me like a good rationale for giving echinacea a try no matter what kind of yeast infection you're dealing with.

★★★ **Foil the offending fungi with garlic.** Garlic is well-known as an antibacterial antibiotic, but it also inhibits fungi quite well and can be used to treat both vaginal candidiasis and thrush. The typical oral dose may range up to a dozen raw, chopped cloves taken two or three times a day in juice. You have to like the taste of garlic pretty much to live with this particular treatment, but I think it's worth a try, as garlic does pack a powerful anti-yeast wallop. (Try blending it with carrots; it's surprisingly easy to take that way.) Onions have a similar but less potent effect.

★★ **Stock up on cranberries.** Arbutin, a compound found in cranberries (and bearberries and blueberries), helps treat candida infections, according to naturopaths Joseph Pizzorno, N.D., president of Bastyr University in Seattle, and Michael Murray, N.D., authors of *A Textbook of Natural Medicine*. So if you're thinking of taking garlic, why not take it with cranberry juice? Or just eat some cranberry sauce plain. These colorful berries are not just for Thanksgiving.

Index

Boldface page references indicate primary discussions.